Jun 2019

Praise for *Aly's Fight*

"In *Aly's Fight*, Josh and Aly reveal how life can be full of interruptions and pain, yet with trust and insistent faith, God crafts the miraculous. *Aly's Fight* is a must-read to the very end. We believe their story will change hearts and stir up faith for those walking through a difficult season."

—**Marcus and Joni Lamb**, Founders of Daystar Television network

"Such a great read! I couldn't put it down. *Aly's Fight* is incredibly encouraging and inspiring!"

—**Margot Ardoin**, Christian, wife,
co-owner of Purposed Communications

"Hope is rare in today's dark world. But Josh and Aly Taylor inspire all of us to hold onto hope and fight with all we have to get to the light without fear."

—**Sadie Robertson**, *New York Times* best-selling author of
Live Original and *Live Fearless*, Founder of LiveOriginal.com

"Josh and Aly tell their story filled with disappointments, highs and lows, and amazing miracles. Their story will give you courage to press on, to never let go of hope, and to stay anchored to the one who will not disappoint you—Jesus Christ."

—**Mac and Mary Owen**, Celebrate Recovery National Directors

"Aly and Josh's joy is palpable in the midst of the hardships they detail as they share the goodness of the Father. Their story is a true testament to the Lord working all things together for good as we are called according to His purposes."

—**Kelly Gonzales**, believer, wife, mother,
Head of School of Agape School of Baton Rouge

"I've had the great privilege of watching Josh and Aly's story unfold before my very eyes. What amazes me the most is even though I have walked alongside them through this journey, every single time I hear their story, it stirs something deep inside of me and it is as if I am hearing it for the very first time."

—**Julie Brown**, believer, wife, and mom

"*Aly's Fight* will keep you at the edge of your seat as you sit on the front row watching Aly and Josh's story unfold. This amazing couple gives all the glory to God and has found hope and restoration that can only come through Jesus Christ."

—**Joe White**, President of Kanakuk Kamps

"Wow! Talk about a roller-coaster ride through life! Aly and Josh Taylor have been through it all—the good, the bad, the wonderful, and the devastating. This book is filled with encouragement, gut-wrenching honesty, humor, and unshakable hope. It is in no way a downer! No matter what you're facing *Aly's Fight* will help keep you in the fight. One of the most uplifting books I've read."

—**Martha Bolton**, Emmy-nominated former staff writer for Bob Hope, and author of 89 books, including *Josiah for President* and *Forgettable Jokes for Older Folks*

"Josh and Aly share real-life faith in the midst of life-changing circumstances. Their story offers hope, real help, and healing to those facing cancer, infertility, or any other unexpected enemy. Their story is a testimony that Jesus is alive and is still working wonders in and among His people. I was greatly encouraged to hear how their faith community came together to help meet every physical, emotional, and spiritual need that arose. What a glorious picture of the body of Christ!"

—**Katy Bolls**, Bible teacher, speaker, joyful mother of children

"This is a life changing book. Josh and Aly share their highest highs and lowest lows, but never once are they without hope. You will be inspired by this uplifting and important book."

—**Korie Robertson**, Star of A&E's, *Duck Dynasty* and *New York Times* best-selling author

"Authentic—that is what I have always known Josh and Aly Taylor to be. Having known both of them most of my life, I can attest that *Aly's Fight* is such an accurate glimpse into this admirable quality they both possess. You are sure to be encouraged as Aly and Josh walk you through the highlights and darkest valleys of their life—a journey marked with love, humor, heartache, miracles and God given joy. Sharing God's story never gets old, this is a MUST READ!"

—**C. Ainsley Beeman**, Christ-follower, co-owner of Purposed Communications

"Reading Josh and Aly's book inspires us and fills our hearts with faith and love for our Father in heaven. After all the struggles and trials, you see that God truly is with us, and has something so beautiful in store for each and every one of us. Our trials prepare us for our greatest successes. Josh and Aly's story is proof of that!"

—**Ashley and Tyson Gardner**, YouTube Family Vloggers @gardnerquadsquad, and Reality Stars of TLC's *Rattled*

"You will be filled with hope and a deeper faith as you read about a God who weaved together Aly and Josh's incredible story and know the same God is weaving your story too."

—**Valerie Woerner**, author of *Grumpy Mom Takes a Holiday* and Owner of Val Marie Paper

"This book is an amazing testament to our amazing God!"

—**Amy Harris**, Worship leader, boy mom

"What an amazing life story, and it's still in its beginning stages! Josh and Aly have fought their many battles with more faith than most can muster. While reading the book I continually heard Exodus 14:14 ringing in my ears, 'The LORD will fight for you, you need only to be still.' Josh and Aly exemplified this verse so well throughout their many, many challenges."

—**Lori Phelps**, Owner of David Phelps Concerts, The Barn @ The Phelps Farm, Barn and Bale

"We love this beautiful family! With six miracle babies of our own, we are truly inspired by Aly and Josh's story of hope and trusting God through the hardest of times."

—**Danielle and Adam Busby**, Reality Stars from TLC's *Outdaughtered*, Founder of ItsABuzzWorld.com

"Great spiritual encouragement to anyone who has a family member dealing with cancer! It is an encouragement to anyone."

—**Jill May**, wife, mom, and counselor

"When we think of curse words, the first word that comes to mind is not usually the "C" word. But for those who have been cursed by cancer, it is much worse than those offensive names and "curses" used to hurt people. Aly and Josh met this hated and dreadful word with the full armor of Christ. Were they afraid? Yes. Were their lives altered? Yes. Did God restore to them a different dream, journey and life? Absolutely yes! God is faithful through every hardship, challenge, loss, death, and life! Read *Aly's Fight* and let them show you through their "c" walk what our amazing God does when we trust in Him."

—**Al and Lisa Robertson**, Authors and Speakers

Aly's Fight

BEATING CANCER,
BATTLING INFERTILITY,
AND BELIEVING IN MIRACLES

ALY AND JOSH TAYLOR

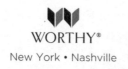

WORTHY®

New York • Nashville

Worthy
Hachette Book Group
1290 Avenue of the Americas, New York, NY 10104
worthypublishing.com
twitter.com/worthypub

First Edition: May 2019

Worthy is a division of Hachette Book Group, Inc. The Worthy name and logo are trademarks of Hachette Book Group, Inc.

The publisher is not responsible for websites (or their content) that are not owned by the publisher.

The Hachette Speakers Bureau provides a wide range of authors for speaking events. To find out more, go to www.hachettespeakersbureau.com or call (866) 376-6591.

Published in association with John Howard, West Monroe, LA.

Cover design by Matt Smartt, Smartt Guys Design
Author photo by Angela Groce, Unveiled Radiance
Print book interior design by Bart Dawson

Library of Congress Cataloging-in-Publication Data

Names: Taylor, Aly (Alyssa Page), 1987- author. | Taylor, Josh, author.
Title: Aly's fight : beating cancer, battling infertility, and believing in miracles / Aly and Josh Taylor.
Description: First edition. | New York : Worthy, 2019.
Identifiers: LCCN 2019004893 | ISBN 9781683972990 (hardcover)
Subjects: LCSH: Taylor, Aly (Alyssa Page), 1987- | Taylor, Josh. | Breast—Cancer—Patients—United States—Biography. | Adoptive parents—United States—Biography.
Classification: LCC RC280.B8 T42 2019 | DDC 362.19699/4490092 [B]—dc23
LC record available at https://lccn.loc.gov/2019004893

ISBNs: 978-1-68397-299-0 (hardcover), 978-1-68397-214-3 (e-book)

Printed in the United States of America
LSC-C
10 9 8 7 6 5 4 3 2 1

This book is dedicated to the most incredible three girls on the planet: our daughters, Genevieve, Vera, and Lydia Taylor. When we look at your faces, we see the heart of God. If we ever question God's goodness, all we have to do is look at you, and all doubts are gone.

Genevieve—you are our reminder of God still being a God of miracles.
Vera—you are our reminder of God doing the impossible.
Lydia—you are our reminder of God's incredible faithfulness to us.

You three girls are chosen, loved, and adored. We are *completely* obsessed with you.

Our greatest prayer and desire for your lives is that you love the Lord your God with all your heart, soul, mind, and strength. Our next prayer is that you love others as you love yourself. You are so incredibly special. We know God will use you all in amazing ways for His kingdom.

God started an incredible work in you from day one of your lives. We are incredibly honored to have a front-row seat to watching how He will complete the work He has begun in you. Love Him. Trust Him. Love others.

Mommy and Daddy love you forever.

— — —

We also want to share a tribute to Aly's dad, Fred Page.

Daddy, you are missed every single day. How I wish you would be sharing in the joys of life in this current season. I know my girls would just adore you the way I still do. I pray we are making you so proud. I cannot wait to jump into your arms in the presence of our Creator and Healer.

I love you always, Aly.

I shall not die, but live,
And declare the works of the LORD.
—Psalm 118:17 (NKJV)

CONTENTS

INTRODUCTION

It has been on our hearts to write this book for years, and we are incredibly humbled to have been given this opportunity to share our story with you.

—ALY—

One day soon after I was first diagnosed with breast cancer, I found myself sitting in the café section of Books-A-Million wanting some time to be quiet and to simply be alone. I was hoping to have time to pray and read. I wanted to get away for a bit from all of the people asking questions about my diagnosis. Everyone was incredibly kind, but all the attention was overwhelming at times.

Lucky for me (insert sarcasm), I had apparently picked the day Paula Deen was doing a book signing, and everyone and their momma was there. We live in West Monroe, Louisiana—a small country town where not many authors, let alone Paula Deen, come for a book signing. What were the chances? I had been in the bookstore for only ten minutes before the crowds started clawing their way in.

As I sat in my chair at the front in the café section and the people started lining up, I started to panic. The last thing I wanted was for anyone to see me. It seemed as if everyone in town knew my news. I was the poor twenty-four-year-old girl who had just been diagnosed with an aggressive form of breast cancer.

To avoid having to talk to anyone, I started walking up and down book aisles in the back. I wanted to stay away from everything cancer related, as I was still in a state of denial, but guess where I ended up—in the aisle with books about cancer.

Despite my reservations, I found myself picking up a few books in this section that looked "faith-based," written by other women who had walked through breast cancer. I started skimming one book written by a woman with a similar type of breast cancer that I had. As I was somewhat enjoying relating to this woman, I got to a part in her book that made me physically ill. She was explaining a hopeful moment in her journey where she learned that there was a high possibility she would live for five years after diagnosis. She was saying that to be encouraging, as this type of cancer was extremely aggressive, and she didn't know if she would have that long.

I got the biggest pit in my stomach. If that statistic held true for me, that would mean I would live until I was twenty-nine! I immediately put the book down. How was that news supposed to be encouraging? I later learned that this girl had been told she only had a few months to live, and she had made it five years. So while she had lived longer that she'd hoped, it was not what I needed to read.

As Paula Deen (finally) left and the crowd dissipated some, I resettled in a chair back in the café section and decided to look up my type of cancer on my computer (you know that was a bad idea) and was met with more horrifying information. I immediately determined that I would stop looking up information or books on my type of cancer because everything was negative. Everything.

I prayed right then and there in that bookstore and said, *Lord, when I am healed . . . not if, but when, I am writing a book that someone can pick up and only be given hope.*

Well, here I am. Writing the book I promised I would write. Praise my Healer and my Sustainer, through cancer, infertility, adoption, pregnancy, and writing this book!

—JOSH—

Aly and I are two ordinary people who have asked God to use us. I think many people say they want to be used by God, but it is another thing to say yes to Him when the circumstances are trying and scary. The song lyric from "Oceans (Where Feet May Fail)" by Hillsong United, "Lead me where my trust is without borders" makes me ponder if I really mean those words when I say them. When I think about those lyrics, my flesh wants to scream (and has screamed), "No, do not lead me where my trust is without borders! Keep me in an easy, safe, enjoyable life where I don't have to trust You much at all." That is just the honest truth.

But the harsh reality is that in this life we will have trouble. As much as we don't want to struggle in life, we will.

And you will too.

We live in a fallen world. So instead of praying for a simple, easy life, I have chosen to embrace the troubles we go through and hold the hand of the One who has overcome them. When we do this, we are living the rich and satisfying life Jesus talks about. Joy in trial. Intimacy with Christ. Peace that surpasses understanding. Let John 16:33 be an anthem whenever you find yourself starting to dwell on the darkness in the world, "I have told you these things, so that in me you may have peace. In this world you will have trouble. But take heart! I have overcome the world."

—JOSH AND ALY—

So here we are. We are Josh and Aly Taylor. We are simply sharing our story and praying that our story impacts yours. We truly believe that many people give up in life right before their breakthrough. Most of our breakthroughs came right after contemplating giving up. Thank God we pushed through, depending on the Lord for our every breath. We pray that reading our story of heartbreak and deliverance will encourage you to keep holding on, and keep believing that God is who He says He is. He will come through for you, in His timing and in His perfect way.

We pray that wherever you are in life, and whoever you are, this book will impact you. We are not special, and our words are not special. But the God who has crafted the most beautiful story in our lives *is*. He is waiting for you to trust Him and completely surrender this crazy, unpredictable life to Him. Want to know how? Come along with us, and we hope that as you read of our complete surrender, you will join us as we choose to live a life surrendered.

CHAPTER 1

WHEN CANCER ~~INTERRUPTED~~ DESTROYED OUR LIFE PLAN

—JOSH AND ALY—

Our lives stopped on October 17, 2011.

Most people have a date in their heads that marks a key change in their lives. A defining moment that gives context to a person's life story. Maybe it was a wedding, a first kiss, the birth of a child, or a new job. For us, that date is October 17, 2011. No matter what the future holds, we know we will always look back on the events of our lives as *pre-October 17* and *post-October 17*. Everything we had ever been, known, thought, hoped for, or dreamed of before that day came to a screeching halt, and an entirely new life we never expected began. God had much bigger and better plans for us than we ever could have imagined; we just had to go through our worst nightmares to get there.

Our story has been equal parts joy, anxiety, hilarity, pain, excitement, and heartbreak. People tell us all the time that we've experienced more life in our first thirty-something years than most people ever do. And with all we've been through, it can be hard to figure out where to even begin telling our story. So we'll start with *us*. This is a story about two people who are deeply in love and absolutely crazy about each other—but it didn't start out that way.

YOUNG LOVE . . . KIND OF

—ALY—

I met Josh Taylor when I was fourteen years old and he was seventeen. Even at that young age, I'd already been through a terrible tragedy. My father—my rock and my hero—had died a few years earlier in a car accident. I remember hearing about my dad's accident and thinking he'd just broken a few bones; I never even considered the possibility that he could be gone. I was making him a get-well card when my mom walked in to tell my sister and me that he had passed away. I was shocked and started screaming, "NO! NO! NOOOO!" Even now, as an adult, I have a hard time comprehending his death. It was the first time in my life when I longed for heaven, knowing that only there will the heartache on earth make sense. Oh, how I wanted to see my daddy again!

As our family was trying to get used to life without him, we moved from my hometown of Lafayette to Monroe, Louisiana. I was enrolled in a local Christian school and was blessed with some new, wonderful friends there. During my freshman year of high school, one of those friends invited me to a party at another student's house. It was there that I saw Josh Taylor for the first time. He was *super* cute in his baggy Abercrombie jeans, and he had a head full of poufy, curly black hair. But he also had an inaccurate reputation for being a bit of a player. We locked eyes a couple of times, and then I saw him heading my way. I remember thinking, *Don't do it. Don't do it. I'm not into you. Please don't do this.*

He did it.

—JOSH—

I grew up as a pastor's kid in West Monroe. From prekindergarten on, I was a student at the small Christian school at my dad's church. Between school, church, and family, I was on the church grounds 24-7. Both my parents worked there, and all my friends were there. I lived and breathed Family

Church and Claiborne Christian School; it was my whole world—and I loved it. Then, as I finished my eighth-grade year, that part of my world was shattered when I found out the school was closing. I'd never even thought about any other school, so I didn't know what that meant for me. My fourteen-year-old brain was overrun with questions like, *Where will I go?* and *What about my friends?* To make matters worse, the school closed because of financial reasons and, well, did I mention both my parents worked there? We moved into a trailer on the church property and did everything we could to cut costs.

I was scared, and everything I'd ever known had changed. When it was time to start high school, my parents decided to send my brother and me to a different Christian school about thirty minutes from our house. Thirty minutes doesn't seem like much now, but at the time I felt like I was being shipped off to another country. Thankfully, some of my best friends decided to go to that school, too, but many others didn't. I was devastated as I started high school and had to build a new life practically from scratch.

Fast-forward two years. My high school didn't seem so new and different anymore. I'd made a pretty good life there, and I had made some great friends. One night at a friend's party, I noticed a stunning beauty across the room. I didn't know much about Aly at the time, only that she was a freshman and seemed like a fun person to be around. And, of course, that she was incredibly beautiful. I know Aly considers that to be her "ugliest phase of life," but I'm here to tell you fourteen-year-old Aly *rocked* some straight-across bangs and braces! My mind was made up. I was going in, and I wasn't coming back without that girl's phone number.

—ALY—

"Do you want to go see a movie with me Sunday?"

Wait, what? Did this "player" really just stroll up to me and ask me out? I was thinking, *I'm not interested! Why are you doing this?* But those weren't the words that came out of my mouth. I was young, and I had never been asked out before. Rather than telling him to take a hike, I heard myself answer, "Sure! Sounds great!"

So two days later, Josh Taylor picked me up for my first date *ever*. Fortunately for us, we have it all documented, thanks to my sister. She filmed and interviewed me as I got ready using her finest fake British accent. I guess you could say that was my first—but certainly not my last—taste of reality television. We've probably watched and laughed at that video a thousand times over the years. My favorite part is the image of Josh driving me away from our house. As the car disappears down the street, my sister jokes, "Well, let's hope we see Aly again!"

Josh was really sweet on that date and did his best to make a good impression, but I just wasn't into him at all. I felt weird and awkward the whole time. I leaned as far away from him as my seat would allow during the movie, terrified he'd try to hold my hand or put his arm around me. When he took me home, I walked in and breathed a huge sigh of relief, grateful the whole ordeal was over. But then he started calling. A lot. I never answered the phone; instead, I armed my mom and sister with a list of excuses to give him for why I couldn't talk. I just couldn't bear to tell him the truth: that we were *never* going out again. Surely he'd get the hint, right?

Wrong. He kept calling! It's crazy that he seemed to believe every awful excuse we gave him. While I wasn't talking to him on the phone, my mom was. And she loved him and felt so bad for him! He and my mom built a lifelong friendship from all those phone conversations he had with her while I was hiding from him!

Finally, I got the nerve to tell him I couldn't date him. I said it was because he was too old. Yes, it was a lie, but I was trying to let him down easily. I should have been honest, though, because my "too old" excuse fell apart a few weeks later when I started dating a guy who was even *older* than Josh. He definitely got the message at that point.

Why did I torture the poor boy? Obviously I had no clue how amazing he was—or what kindness hid beneath that pouf of curly hair. Thank goodness time has a way of changing hearts, minds, and hairstyles. With time and perspective, Jesus can help us see that our young, immature thoughts can be pretty silly. It won't surprise you to hear that about a year later I realized how much of a mistake I'd made in letting Josh go.

During lunch at school one day, I was eyeballing Josh as he laughed with one of his friends, and I commented to a friend that he was really cute. I had learned that he wasn't the "player" I'd assumed he was; he was just fun and made people smile. It's amazing what a year and a good haircut can do! My friend, the teenage girl that she was, decided to play the role of matchmaker and tell Josh I was interested in him.

Now, let me tell you something about Josh Taylor: he doesn't waste any time. When he sees something he wants, he goes for it! So almost immediately after my friend talked to him, he came right up to me and asked me out. That date—and every date afterward—went *much* differently than our first one did. I will always be thankful that he wanted me enough to pursue me *twice*.

—JOSH—

Yes, Aly finally came to her senses! I was so embarrassed when she ditched me the year before and was understandably leery when her friend told me she was suddenly into me. I had a bruised ego and did not want a repeat of the previous year's fiasco, but it was a risk worth taking. I knew there was something special about this girl. Even if I only had a slim chance of winning her over, I *had* to take it. Fortunately, things worked out *much* better for us this time around.

Aly was different from any girl I'd ever known. The truth is, she was downright intimidating. There's one image in my mind in particular that sums up who she is, even when she was a teenager. Shortly after we began dating, she and I went on a group ski trip together. Technically she was there with her girlfriends and I was there with my guy friends. Our relationship was new, and we were still getting to know each other, but that trip told me everything I needed to know about her.

One night Aly excused herself from the group to go to bed early. A little while later, I went upstairs to get something out of my room, and I noticed that the door to the girls' room was open. As I walked past, I saw Aly sitting up and studying her Bible. Every other teenager in the building was either talking, playing, or sleeping, but there was Aly, reading her Bible and spending time alone with the Lord. To be honest, I probably didn't even *pack* a Bible for that trip, but Aly made Bible study a priority even during spring break. I went to bed that night thinking, *Am I out of my league?* The answer, of course, was yes—but I didn't let that stop me. I wasn't about to let her slip away again.

Somehow I managed not to blow it, and Aly and I fell madly in love. We all hear about how young love isn't *real* and how two people need to grow up and figure out who they are as individuals before they make big decisions about the person they are going to spend their life with. I totally get that, and I know a lot of young people make a ton of stupid decisions they later regret. However, even if it's a one-in-a-million chance, young love can be a beautiful type of love. Being able to grow up with my wife has been one of the most amazing gifts of my life. I was with Aly when she got her driver's license. We celebrated each other's high school graduation. We moved each other in and out of dorms and apartments. We have a shared history of life experience at the heart of our relationship. Most importantly, we have seen each other at our best and worst in the past fifteen years, and we have seen God sustain us no matter what's come our way. And, as you'll see, we've been through a lot.

BUILDING A LIFE TOGETHER

—ALY—

Even though we began our relationship when we were young, Josh and I haven't been joined at the hip every day since that first (well, technically *second*) date. After high school, we lived in different cities, with me at LSU and Josh figuring out what he wanted to do with his life. That time apart only clarified what we thought God was telling us: that we were meant to spend the rest of our lives together. We knew we were ready to commit our lives to each other forever, and we wanted *forever* to start as soon as possible. So, on July 22, 2006, at the ages of 21 and 19, Josh Taylor and Aly Page tied the knot and started a crazy adventure together.

We had a huge wedding with more than seven hundred friends and family members celebrating with us. Because we'd been together so long, our families were already close and practically all our friends were *our* friends. We were part of an amazing community, and our wedding was a celebration of that wonderful, gigantic family of believers. We had no idea then how important that history and support system would become.

We spent the next five years doing typical newlywed and young adult stuff. We moved around a few times as Josh got his career off the ground. It was a little bumpy at times, but overall, it was five years of marital bliss. I'm definitely the planner of the family, so any little *surprises* made me tweak what Josh and I called "my plan." The plan was simple: move closer to our parents, work and save for a couple more years, do some traveling, and try to start having children when I was around twenty-three because I wanted to be a young mom. Then we'd get a nicer house, move up the corporate ladder, and raise some awesome kids. You know, typical American dream stuff.

While Josh did some experimenting to figure out what he wanted to do professionally, I always knew what I wanted to do—be a mom. This was always the biggest desire of my heart after being a wife, so I never spent much time dreaming about careers. However, while in college, God put marriage and family therapy on my heart and I decided to pursue that field of study. Although I always desired to be a homemaker and be with my future kids as much as possible, I knew that learning more about marriage and family would not only be a precursor to my possible future employment, but it would help me in my own marriage and with our future children. Two birds, one stone!

I started a master's program so I could start a family therapy career. The plan was for me to work for a while until we had our first child. I'd stay home with the kids until they were in school. Then I could go back to work if I wanted to. I was excited about helping other marriages, families, and children, but I was *more* excited about raising my children. I couldn't wait to meet them!

—JOSH—

Our first few years of marriage were indeed amazing, and despite walking through a few relocations, a job loss, school, and financial worries, we enjoyed the life we were building together. We were—and are—such great partners.

By our fifth wedding anniversary, I was working as the director of development and basketball coach at a private school, and Aly had started a PhD program in marriage and family therapy. For a little more excitement, we decided to build our first home too. Life for us as a couple was coming together, and soon it would be time for the next step on Aly's life plan: babies!

When Aly mentioned being ready to start a family, though, I sensed a surprising restlessness stirring inside of me. I felt unsettled at my core, and I believed God was telling me to quit the coaching portion of my job. I spent so many nights thinking and praying, *What? Why? How could this make sense right now?* The team had just come off one of the most successful seasons in the school's history, we were building a house, and we were about to start a family. How in the world would it make sense for me to give up a significant portion of our income?

I knew I would be crushing Aly's dreams, but I had to tell her what I was feeling. It was a hard conversation, but Aly supported me. She said I needed to follow my convictions and trust that those convictions were from the Holy Spirit. I would still have my job at the school as the director of development, and, I reasoned, I could save money on the house by doing some of the work myself with the extra time I'd free up. While I wasn't being completely financially irresponsible, it was definitely a risk. That didn't scare me since I am the risk-taker, but Aly likes predictability. I realized this decision was stretching her, which made me even more grateful for her support.

After more prayer and seeking wise counsel from a mentor, I quit my coaching job. As soon as I did, I felt an immediate rush of peace about it. It was hard for others to understand, especially with no real concrete reason for quitting other than feeling directed by God to do so, but I knew without a doubt this was the right move for our family. It's often hard for Christians to decipher what messages come from the Holy Spirit and what messages come from our own minds, but I knew this was a Holy Spirit calling. I also believe our obedience to God's call on our lives always leads to a fuller life in Christ—even when the road ahead takes you on some terrifying twists and turns that you never saw coming. I didn't know it at the time, but God was freeing up my time for some important work that was just around the corner. He truly goes before us and prepares the way.

EVERYTHING CHANGES

—ALY—

I was scared when Josh quit his coaching job, but he and I were both convinced it was the right decision—even though we didn't know *why* it was the right decision. And to add to the craziness, we decided we'd start trying to get pregnant. We were living with his parents at the time, we were building a house, Josh was reexamining his career, and I was starting my PhD program. In many ways, this didn't seem like the best time to grow our family. As we continued to talk, though, we agreed there would *never* be a perfect time. There would always be something to worry about, so we figured this was as good a time as any. As it turned out, the timing actually *was* perfect—just not in the way we expected.

Josh and I saved ourselves sexually for marriage, but as a young woman, I had still spent years and years hearing all the lectures and warnings about preventing pregnancy. By the time we abandoned our birth control methods and started trying to have a child, I was convinced we'd get pregnant the first try. That didn't happen. Apparently my body didn't get the memo about my life plan. The first month went by, then the second. No baby. After the second month of trying, I burst into tears when I saw the negative pregnancy test result. I couldn't help but think, *What's wrong with me?* You may laugh at me for breaking down after only two months, especially if you've been through the struggles of infertility yourself, but I didn't know then what I know now. I had never even considered the possibility of not getting pregnant.

At one point I thought, *The test result is wrong. I know I'm pregnant. I can feel it.* That's right, regardless of the unmistakable negative line on the test, I convinced myself I was pregnant. I mean, I had all these symptoms. *Something* had to be going on with me. I consulted the world's greatest medical expert, Google, and searched for signs of pregnancy. Nausea? Check! Weird appetite? Check! Strange bowel movements? Gross, but check! Late period? Check! Sore breasts? Hmm. I wasn't sure. Maybe they were, but that usually happened near my period anyway. I decided to jump in the shower and do a breast self-exam, trying to convince myself that my breasts were sore. Well, they weren't. But I did notice something; I felt a little lump in my breast. I wondered if the lump meant that my milk was coming in because I was pregnant. Laugh if you want. I was working toward a PhD, not an MD!

The lump got my attention, though. I got out of the shower and had Josh feel it. He and I both thought it was nothing dangerous, but we agreed I would get it looked at. Better safe than sorry, right?

—JOSH—

I really didn't think that little knot in her breast was a big deal, but I wanted to support her in getting anything checked out that concerned her. She saw the doctor and then had an ultrasound done. They said it was likely a fibroadenoma, a benign lump, and we decided to have it removed.

We were all relieved when Aly got out of surgery, and the surgeon said he was 99.9 percent sure it was indeed a fibroadenoma. He explained that this was common in young women and told us to go home and rest in peace knowing all was well. On our way home from the hospital, we discussed how thankful we were to already have a reasonably final diagnosis instead of having to wait a few days. I commented on how differently the day could have gone if we had gotten bad news instead. It was another day of praise for the Taylor family!

At church the following Sunday, I felt a strong urge to have Aly go down for prayer with the elders. She gave me a strange look when I mentioned it, clearly not understanding why. I said something about not being able to explain the feeling, and she agreed to have the elders pray over her. I'm not saying I knew something was wrong; I didn't. I just knew God was calling me to cover my wife in prayer. None of us knew that the following day would change our lives forever.

—ALY—

The next day was—you guessed it—October 17, 2011. We already told you our lives changed forever that day, so you can probably guess what happened.

I knew a nurse would call with the official results from my biopsy that day, but I wasn't concerned. The doctor told us it was nothing. Just a benign little knot. Certainly nothing worth worrying about. Josh and I went about our day like normal and drove to the house we were building to work for the afternoon. After a couple of hours sanding baseboards and filling holes with putty, my phone rang, and I saw that it was the doctor's office. I answered, expecting the friendly nurse to be on the other end. Instead, it was the surgeon who had reassured me that everything was fine just a couple of days earlier. Any optimism he'd had in his voice the last time we'd talked was gone.

"Aly," he said with a nervous crack in his voice. "I am so shocked, but your biopsy results came back . . . and it is breast cancer."

I don't remember anything else he said after that, but I will never forget those words. The words that changed my life forever. The words that I feared would *end* my life.

It was supposed to be so simple: young love, happy marriage, career, children, health, and happiness. I was twenty-four years old. This was supposed to be the time in our lives when a doctor was calling to tell us I was pregnant. But it wasn't a baby growing inside my body; it was cancer. My plan was ruined.

CHAPTER 2

BREAST CANCER AT TWENTY-FOUR?!

—JOSH—

Aly's cries echoed through our empty, unfinished home as she slid down the wall and collapsed onto the bare floor. She wrapped her arms around her chest—which was still bandaged from the biopsy surgery—and screamed, "God! Heal me! Please! Please heal me, God!"

I ran over and fell on the floor next to her. "What is it? What's going on?" I asked, but she couldn't tell me. She was just weeping and weeping. Her face was completely white; I'd never seen that look in the eight years I'd known her. I knew I'd heard the words *breast cancer*, but that didn't make any sense. Aly had always been ridiculously healthy. Seriously, the girl never got sick. Besides, the doctor had told us days earlier that there was nothing to worry about, and now they were talking about cancer? No way. At worst, I thought she might have just *a little bit* of cancer. Is that even a thing?

As she sat balled up in the corner of the room crying and praying, I grabbed the telephone. I needed answers. I'm her husband; I fix things. How could I fix this if I didn't know what was going on? So I called the doctor back to make sure Aly had heard correctly. Surely she'd misunderstood.

The doctor answered the phone himself; it had probably only been thirty seconds since he'd hung up with Aly. I blurted out, "Is it true? Does my wife really have cancer?"

"Yes, Josh. I'm so sorry, but she does." His tone left no doubt, but just to drive the point home, he told me this was a very serious situation. He wanted to meet us in his office the following day to discuss our next steps.

What do you say in that situation? Arguing with the doctor wouldn't help, and the terror and frustration left me speechless. There was nothing I could do to fix this. I hung up and fell on the floor next to my wife. Only moments before, we were goofing off and sanding baseboards in our new home; now we were crying and praying for God to save her life.

We are all truly one phone call away from falling to our knees.

WHAT NOW?

—ALY—

That afternoon, before the phone call that changed everything, Josh and I were laughing and joking about our future. There was no doubt we'd be pregnant soon, and we decided the very room we were sanding could be the baby's nursery. I came up with a great idea: We'd paint "Baby's Room" on the walls before we finished painting everything. Then we could bring our parents over for a tour of our in-progress home. When they got to this room, they'd see "Baby's Room" and know we were pregnant! What a celebration that would be! Everyone would be so happy; it would be a day we'd always remember.

That vision was fresh in my mind as the phone rang. Literally one minute I was dreaming about our pregnancy reveal and the next I was on the floor crying, praying, and wondering if I would ever be able to have children—if I lived at all. Talk about a whirlwind.

I've often wondered how people get through life without a saving relationship with Jesus Christ. This was one of those times. The only—and I mean *only*—thing I had hope in during this moment was that I had Jesus living in me, and I truly believed He could heal me. But what would it look like to walk out that faith in real life? I didn't even know what to do for the rest of that afternoon and night. I mean, I knew we were meeting with the doctor the next day, but what should we do in the meantime? I thought, *Do we keep sanding the room? Do we leave? Who should we call? How am I going to sleep tonight? Do we go to work and school in the morning?* We were clueless.

As I sat there feeling overwhelmed, Matthew 6:34 came to mind: "Therefore do not worry about tomorrow, for tomorrow will worry about itself. Each day has enough trouble of its own." I knew if I thought too far into the future I would become extremely overwhelmed and caught up in worry. I had to focus on today. *Today I learned I had cancer.* I felt as though the world should stop for a while to let me adjust, but I realized a hard truth about life: it goes on. The world doesn't stop spinning, not even long enough for a twenty-four-year-old girl to deal with the worst news she could imagine.

—JOSH—

After a long time curled on the unfinished floor, Aly and I got up and drove back to my parents' house. We were staying there while we built our house, but they were out of town that night. Aly's mom and several of our friends met us there to show their love and support as the diagnosis sank in. None of us could believe it, and none of us knew how to act. I knew Aly was struggling, and I did everything I could to support her. But the truth is, I was falling apart inside. I wanted to be her rock, but I was crumbling. At some point denial crept in and I told myself it wasn't as bad as we were making it out to be. I even let myself sneak off to a far part of the house and hang out with my lifelong friend Kyle for a little while. Everything was surreal, and I think I was trying to establish some sort of normalcy.

After everyone went home, Aly and I were left in the big house all alone. We went to bed and held hands in silence as we each tried to get some sleep. Weird thoughts kept running through my head. *Will she be sicker when she wakes up? Is cancer noticeably worse every day?* We were so clueless.

We got up the following morning and weren't sure what to do. We knew we couldn't go to work or school, but Aly's appointment wasn't until 2:00 p.m. We took a long morning walk, but neither of us said much. Our phone rang every two minutes with a friend or family member checking in. They asked a million questions, but we didn't have any answers. All we could do was wait until the doctor's appointment and pray for the doctor to tell us a single, simple surgery would take care of the problem once and for all. I think we both just wanted to get past this little bump in the road as quickly as possible so we could get on with our lives.

—ALY—

My doctor's appointment was a wake-up call. Josh and I had been trying to convince ourselves that even though it was cancer, this wouldn't be a big deal. The look on my doctor's face was all it took to crush that hope. It's a terrifying thing to see fear in your doctor's eyes, but there it was. He was kind and compassionate, but there was no small talk; he was all business. He ran through the biopsy test results and mentioned different numbers and statistics, but it basically came down to this: I definitely had cancer, and it was extremely aggressive—actually, the *most* aggressive type of breast cancer. Things just kept getting worse.

My list-making, action-oriented brain sprung to life, and I hit him with all the questions I could think of about what we should do next. Because of the severity of the cancer, the doctor said he'd only be comfortable if I went to the best cancer hospital around. As qualified as he was, he knew he was out of his depth on this one. He arranged for me to see a specialist at MD Anderson Cancer Center in Houston, Texas, as soon as possible. With that, he wished us well and said goodbye. There was nothing left for us to do except wait and pray—two things I did *not* want to do. I wanted to jump into action, to go to war and all-out attack the enemy in my body, but it wasn't time yet. All I could do was wait and pray. I was devastated, frustrated, and yet still filled with faith and hope. God's presence was still so real in my life, even though everything else seemed to be falling apart.

We drove back to the house in a stunned state of silence. I remember crying on the couch and trying to explain the anxiety I felt at not being able to do anything except wait. Josh, God bless him, told me later that he didn't know what to do at the time. He said he thought of several Bible verses he could have shared, but he chose to simply sit there with me and let me cry on him. That was such the right move. I love that his mind went straight to Scripture, and we've since spent countless hours talking about those verses and what they meant for my recovery, but I didn't need a sermon that day. I needed my husband, and he was there for me. I remember thinking how blessed I was to have such a history with Josh for the fight ahead, as he knew what I needed and when I needed it.

MD Anderson finally called and scheduled my appointment for October 26—nine days after my doctor first said the word *cancer*. Somehow just having that appointment on the calendar helped me relax a little. For the first time I felt like we had some kind of plan, like we were actually *doing something*. Sitting around and waiting was making me physically ill, but those days of waiting and praying were good for me. It was a hard-fought lesson in letting God fight my battles, a lesson I'd have to come back to again and again over the next few years. As Exodus 14:14 says, "The LORD will fight for you; you need only to be still." As hard as it was for me to be still, I knew this was a battle only He could fight—and win—for me.

SHARING OUR STORY

"Look! There are already fifty comments!"

I woke up the next morning to Josh excitedly shoving his laptop in my face. I had no idea what he was talking about, but I hadn't seen him genuinely excited about anything since we got the doctor's first phone call. We were still waiting for our MD Anderson appointment and trying to make the best of each day without driving ourselves (and each other) crazy with worry.

I asked Josh what I was looking at, and he explained that he had started a blog to document my cancer journey. It was his way of keeping everyone informed on what was going on and sharing specific prayer requests. The look on his face was precious. I knew he was expecting a big, sweet "thank you" from me. Instead, I thought I might throw up. I'm a private person by nature. It's hard for me to share intimate details of my life with others, which is ironic considering we're less than two chapters into this book and I've already told you about my breasts, pregnancy tests, and weird bowel movements. Oh, how cancer changes a person!

Back then, though, I felt sick at the thought of the whole world knowing I had cancer. On the other hand, I was grateful for the chance to let people know how they could pray for me. As I struggled with Josh's decision to start a blog, someone shared the phrase "prayers over privacy" with me. That became our family motto for the blog. I knew we needed the body of Christ to cover us in prayer for the journey we were about to take. So I made the willful decision to push aside my need for privacy in order to keep my friends and family informed and to give them the opportunity to pray for our specific needs. I also prayed and trusted that our blog would be a source of inspiration for others.

Josh's first post went online on October 20, 2011—just a few days after we found out I had cancer. I guess he was having a little trouble waiting and praying too. Should he have asked me first? Probably. But then, if he had, I most likely would have said no—and saying no would have prevented us from experiencing one of our biggest blessings throughout the whole cancer ordeal. The blog became a lifeline for us, a place to share our thoughts, prayers, fears, joys, and, in time, our encouragement to others going through the same thing. God has worked miracles in and through that little blog, and I'm so grateful to Josh for creating it. But seriously, babe. Next time, ask!

PARTIES, PRAYERS, AND (FALSE) HOPES

—JOSH—

Aly's cancer hospital was located in Houston, so we knew we'd be on the road a lot for the next several months. The Sunday before we left for that first appointment, our friends Angie and Julie arranged an old-fashioned prayer and encouragement meeting to give us a proper, prayer-filled send-off. There was singing, laughing, prayers, and a ton of food. Sweet friends, Amy and Ron, led worship and sang songs of faith over Aly. At one point Aly had a chance to speak. In what she later described as a "naïve, Holy Spirit bubble," she actually said the words, "I am excited for this journey." I'd seen a lot of emotions over the past week, and *excitement* wasn't one of them. But Aly was doing the best she could in an impossible situation.

As we left the party that night, we talked about how cool it was for Angie and Julie to do that for us. Angie is a leukemia survivor and she and her husband, Richard, became mentors for us as we walked through our own cancer fight. Aly and I decided that after Aly beat this thing, we would open our home like that for others walking through cancer. That, we agreed, is what mentorship is all about—helping others get through something you've been through yourself. And we were *determined* to get through this.

Aly, myself, and Aly's mom, Cyd, hit the road the next morning heading to Houston for the first of what would be many appointments. On the way, we made a pit stop in Baton Rouge to get another opinion from a respected oncologist there. As we walked into that office, Aly was visibly uncomfortable. The cancer patients in the waiting room looked sick. *Is Aly really a cancer patient?* I didn't even know what to call her. I couldn't associate her name with cancer, but I also had to face the reality of the situation. As we waited with the other cancer patients, I realized Aly was now one of them.

When we finally walked into the doctor's office, he was reviewing a sheet with Aly's name on it, but it was spelled "Allie." We told him it was misspelled, and he got a strange look on his face. He looked at the birth-date on the sheet, and it was for a woman born in the 1930s. He was confused and said this was the paperwork that was sent from the doctor who did Aly's biopsy. Suddenly we were given a glimmer of hope. Could what we prayed for be coming to pass? Did the wrong Aly/Allie Taylor get the cancer diagnosis? We prayed, *Please, God, make them realize that the biopsy, the cancer, the severity—everything—was wrong!* The doctor told us not to get too excited, as it probably was just a typo. So we waited. And waited. And waited.

The doctor returned with the correct paperwork, but his dire expression hadn't changed. Despite the mix-up, Aly—*my Aly*—had cancer. After a rush of false hope and what felt like a cruel joke, we were right back where we started. The Baton Rouge doctor echoed everything we'd already heard. He told us Aly would most likely need a mastectomy and additional treatment, but we wouldn't know for sure until more surgeries and scans were done.

Sitting there in that doctor's office, having already been to one doctor and on our way to seeing another, it dawned on me that every doctor might say something different. How would we know which one to trust? How would we know which one had the best plan? What if we screwed up and made the wrong decisions? As these questions were swimming through my head, I had to call a friend—himself a doctor—to ask for a favor. While we were talking he asked me for an update on Aly's situation, and I told him we had stopped for another opinion on the way to Houston.

That call turned out to be crucial in our cancer journey. My friend lovingly but forcefully said, "Josh, if you keep hearing different opinions and don't settle on one, you will drive yourself crazy. You have to choose to follow *one*." He was right. We were surrounding ourselves with experts, and after hearing what the doctors had to say at MD Anderson, it would be time to pick the best course of action using the facts available and the leading of the Holy Spirit. This was a critical reminder for me that I couldn't fix this situation. I couldn't heal Aly; not even the doctors could heal her. Only God and God *alone* could heal His sick child.

A BIRTHDAY BLESSING

—ALY—

We woke up in Houston the next day. My big doctor's appointment was the following day, but *this* day was Josh's twenty-seventh birthday. I love birthdays, and I always go all out on Josh's birthday to make him feel as special and loved as he is. But here I was, waking up out of town and without a gift for my husband. That had never happened in all the years we'd been together.

With no other options, I grabbed a piece of printer paper, folded it in half, and made him a homemade birthday card. I expressed how much I loved him and how sorry I was about him spending his birthday like this. Of course he thought my apology was ridiculous. This was when the guilt process started for me, though. I grew extremely guilty for what Josh was going through and what he was about to encounter. Instead of giving him a baby, I was giving him a nightmare of stress and worry. Time, perspective, and God's grace have given me a different view of things now, but that's where I was in those early days. I loved this man more than anything, and I felt as though I was ruining not only this birthday but his entire life.

—JOSH—

Aly's mom had been with us since the beginning of Aly's diagnosis and here she was with us in Houston too. She offered to take us anywhere I wanted for my birthday. She had come with us so she could go to her daughter's appointment, not to celebrate my birthday, but she still had a way of making me feel special. I chose a nice steakhouse for dinner, and the three of us headed off. I dropped them off at the front of the restaurant while I hunted for a parking spot. Just a few minutes later I walked inside and saw them sitting at a booth. As soon as I got near the table, I saw that it was covered in confetti and Happy Birthday signs. *Oh, these two,* I thought. *I should have known they'd do something for me!* Even with the uncertainty of the next day's appointment hanging in the air, I couldn't help but thank God for the blessings He'd brought into my life.

—ALY—

Here's what Josh didn't realize about his birthday dinner: My mom and I hadn't planned *anything*. No confetti. No signs. Nothing. The hostess at the restaurant showed us to a table as Josh parked the car, and the three of us were surprised to see the table covered in birthday decorations. The hostess said, "Oh, I am so sorry! We just had a birthday celebration in here. I'll have someone come clean it all off for you immediately."

My mom and I, practically in unison, exclaimed, "Don't take it off!" We looked at each other with tears in our eyes, thanking God for this simple sign that He loved us and was there with us. When Josh walked up and saw the table, the look on his face gave me so much joy. I eventually told him that we didn't decorate the table for him, but the truth made the whole thing even more special. We knew it was God who decorated the table that night. He was there in Houston with us, and we were trusting that we would soon have another party to celebrate our victory over cancer. More confetti would be in our future, in Jesus's name.

THE APPOINTMENT

The next day was the day we were both looking forward to and dreading: my first appointment at MD Anderson. A big crowd had joined us in

Houston, as Josh's parents and several friends came to support us and sit with my mom while we were back with the doctors. They weren't the only people there who knew me, though. The entire staff at the hospital already knew all about me; I felt like the most popular patient around. However, while popularity usually has its perks, you *do not* want to be the most popular patient at MD Anderson Cancer Center. If everyone there knows everything about you the day you show up, there's a good chance you're going to be hanging out with those people for a *long* time.

The team told me immediately that I would need additional testing before they could come up with a full treatment plan, but from what they knew from the biopsy, they expected a mastectomy and most likely chemotherapy and radiation. I wasn't sure what all those words meant other than I would lose my hair and my breasts and that I was sick. I quickly underwent lots of tests and was ushered from one room to another for several different appointments. In between, we checked in with our family and had to keep telling them more and more bad news. The day wasn't totally without a little humor, however.

—JOSH—

Aly had about a million different tests and scans that day. After her mammogram, MRI, and CAT scan, she was taken up for a bone scan to see if the cancer had spread to her bones. They sat Aly in a huge mint-green pleather chair as the technician explained the procedure. She was a sweet woman, and it was clear she knew her stuff. However, she had a thick Indian accent, and Aly and I couldn't fully understand everything she was saying. The tech told us they would inject contrast dye into Aly and then Aly could "pee." Aly and I looked at each other, not fully catching what she meant. I repeated, "Aly is going to pee?"

The tech replied, "Yes, go pee. Do not try and hold it. Just let it go."

"Let it go?" I asked. Suddenly it became clear why Aly was sitting in a large pleather chair. Apparently she was going to pee in it as soon as they injected the dye. I thought, *Is this the "pee chair"? How is this okay? And even remotely sanitary?* I am a bit of a germaphobe, but this was crazy. Aly asked me to go get a set of clothes from the car, and we both wondered why no one warned us to bring some clothes she wouldn't mind peeing in. As we were having this conversation, the nurse burst out laughing.

"No, no! You will have an hour from the **time the** dye is administered before the actual bone scan. So if you need to pee during that time, go pee. Don't hold it. But . . . *go in the bathroom.*" Aly and I cracked up. She told me later that she probably would have filled that chair with pee as soon as they injected the dye out of pure placebo effect if they hadn't cleared that up.

It may seem strange to tell such a silly story from what was an altogether terrifying day, but that is a precious memory for us. It was a powerful reminder that God gives us joy and laughter even in the midst of heartache. We get to choose whether we will laugh and smile or become bitter and angry. Aly and I chose joy. We knew there wouldn't be many opportunities to laugh during those days, so when we had the opportunity, we took it.

You may be facing a nightmare of your own right now, and laughing may seem impossible. Give it a try anyway. Embrace the precious moments of levity even when facing extremely devastating times. As the Bible says, "Consider it pure joy, my brothers and sisters, whenever you face trials of many kinds, because you know that the testing of your faith produces perseverance" (James 1:2–3). We considered the joy—because we needed perseverance.

WORSE THAN WE THOUGHT

—ALY—

After the near-miss peeing incident, I was taken for an ultrasound. They were targeting the site where I'd had the lump removed, and they also mentioned wanting to check the lymph nodes. The ultrasound technician and I had a great chat as she performed the scan. It had been a long day, and I was relieved it was almost over. Even though I had an aggressive cancer, I knew we had caught it early—early enough, I hoped, that it hadn't yet spread anywhere else in my body. The relief I felt evaporated when the ultrasound tech's tone and expression abruptly changed. She told me to sit tight for a minute and that the doctor would be in soon. That's never a good sign.

The doctor told me I had several swollen lymph nodes in my armpit. There was a good chance that was caused by the biopsy surgery I'd had a couple of weeks earlier, so they needed to do a quick needle biopsy of the lymph nodes to make sure no cancer cells were present. They took the cells and asked if I wanted Josh to come back to sit with me while I waited for the results. With panic starting to creep in (again), I said yes. Everything was happening so fast; I had a hard time processing it all. Tears were streaming down my face when he walked in. I told him about the swollen lymph nodes and that we had to sit there and wait for yet another biopsy report.

Just five minutes later, the doctor returned with the same expression I had seen on my doctor's face back home nine days earlier. The news wasn't good. She explained that I had cancer in my lymph nodes and that this cancer was far more serious than anyone had previously thought. *What is happening?* I thought. *How could it be more serious than the aggressive cancer they already told me about? What's more serious than the most aggressive kind of breast cancer you can get?*

Everything changed. Again. More appointments were made. More tests were scheduled. They hadn't staged my cancer yet (telling me where I was on the Stage I–IV scale), but any hopes we had for a low-stage diagnosis were out the window—possibly along with our hopes for starting a family. We'd find out for sure the next day.

CHAPTER 3

WALKING OUT HEALING

—JOSH—

"Do you guys want to have children down the road?"

The question hung in the air like a lead balloon. I can still hear the oncologist's exact somber tone as she hit us with that loaded question at the start of what would be an excruciatingly long day.

Aly's ultrasound and biopsy the day before had shown cancer cells in her lymph nodes, and we had spent a mostly sleepless night wondering what this new information meant. When we left the hospital the day before, all we knew was that Aly had cancer, and it had spread from her breast to her lymph nodes. That didn't sound good, but we still clung to the hope that we caught it early enough to cut it out, burn it out, and pray it out without putting her life in even more danger. Those hopes were challenged when the doctor staged Aly's cancer: Stage III.

Ouch. That news hit us pretty hard. Previously the doctors had seemed worried, but we'd been hearing Stage I thrown around loosely. Now things seemed much, much worse. While the doctors confirmed that Aly had caught the cancer early—she probably hadn't had cancer long at all—she had an extremely aggressive form, and it was growing faster than anyone expected.

While we were processing all of this, the oncologist asked us the baby question: "Do you guys want to have children down the road?" The doctor couldn't have known that we had been trying to grow our family for the past few months. She didn't know that's how Aly had discovered the lump in the first place. That lump. Had it really been only a few weeks since she'd found it? So much had changed since she'd stepped out of the shower that day and asked me to feel that little knot in her breast. We had been frustrated about not being pregnant after two months of trying. Now my wife had Stage III breast cancer that was already spreading throughout her body. It was hard to process.

Aly and I shot a look at each other when the doctor asked about having children, and we told her we'd been trying. She listened and then launched into a speech I'm sure she's given to hundreds of couples. She strongly encouraged us to talk to a fertility specialist as soon as possible. Aly's cancer treatment, she explained, would inevitably include an intense cocktail of chemotherapy drugs and radiation that would make a future pregnancy unlikely. It was weird to hear that the drugs used to *save* her life would also prevent us from bringing a *new* life into the world.

The doctor told us about a fertility practice in Houston that specialized in cancer patients. She needed us to let her know immediately if that was something we wanted to pursue, but she at least gave us an hour to talk and pray about it. The bottom line was that if we wanted to have a child with both Aly's DNA and mine, we needed to get a fertility doctor's help as soon as possible. This would delay Aly's cancer treatment for two weeks (which is why the oncologist needed an answer), but it would probably be the only way to ensure we'd be able to have a biological child someday.

NO TIME TO WAIT

—ALY—

Devastated. That's the only word that describes how I felt. Devastated that I had cancer. Devastated that my family was walking through this nightmare with me. Devastated that I had to consider fertility treatments. Devastated that I was about to start cancer treatment. It was all happening so fast. Every time we got one piece of bad news, we barely had time to get our feet back under us before the bottom fell out again with even *more* bad news. It was only through the guidance of the Holy Spirit that we were able to make sense of any of this craziness.

When I was first diagnosed a few weeks earlier, someone made an off-hand comment about fertility options. I had no idea what they were talking about at the time. I remember thinking, *Fertility options? What do you mean? I have cancer; my fertility is fine!* Oh, naïve me.

Josh and I discussed the fertility option with our family in the waiting room, and we were all in agreement. We were going through with the fertility treatments. Sure, it would delay my cancer regimen by two weeks, but it was worth it to protect our future Baby Taylor. As much as we wished we didn't have to have this conversation, it was exciting to think about creating a little Josh or Aly to put inside my body after this cancer ordeal was behind us. It gave us a glimmer of hope and joy that helped us see past the cancer looming over us. Our family prayed with us over this decision, and we felt a peace about it all. Well, for a second or two, anyway.

Our group had barely said "amen" before Josh and I were called back in to see the oncologist. We had my mom come back with us, too, as we knew this conversation would be an important one. I thought, *That was fast. They told us we had an hour to discuss fertility before we had any other tests or appointments.* The oncologist came into the exam room, and Josh and I were ready to tell her that we'd decided to delay the cancer treatment in order to have the fertility preservation procedures. She started talking before we could, though. It was then that I noticed the new stack of papers in her hands and the new look of devastation on her face.

Almost immediately she started apologizing to us. She said she'd just run a new test on the cancer cells they'd removed the previous day. Although she knew I was Stage III and that I had an aggressive form of cancer, even she was shocked at how quickly the cancer was growing. I'm no doctor, and a lot of these things were hard for me to grasp, so she put it in terms we'd understand. She explained that, if you ranked cancer's aggressiveness on a scale of one to one hundred, mine would likely be a ninety-eight. As if that wasn't bad enough on its own, that also meant we couldn't afford to wait two more weeks before starting my cancer treatment. There was no time to preserve my fertility.

Josh and I were shocked, scared, and horrified. I asked, "We can't even wait two more weeks?" I thought (but couldn't say aloud), *Does this mean I'm going to die? And if I don't die, does this mean I'll never be a mother?* I was processing so many emotions at once. The oncologist said the decision to delay treatment was up to us, and we asked her what she would do if this were happening to her daughter. Her words still echo in my head to this day. She said, "If it was my daughter, I would have wanted her to begin treatment *yesterday*." Any flash of joy we'd had in the waiting room talking about Baby Taylor was gone. We were back to life-and-death decisions. Again I prayed, *Jesus, please heal me!*

—JOSH—

The room was spinning. We just kept getting hit by one piece of bad news after another, and Aly and I had to find our footing. I asked the doctor and Aly's mom to leave the room so we could spend a few minutes alone together to pray and process everything. Neither of us spoke much in that moment. This day . . . this week . . . this entire month had been an absolute nightmare, and so much had happened in the past twenty-four hours. Aly and I collapsed into each other. We hugged and wept. We prayed. We asked God to guide us. We begged Him to save Aly's life. We asked Him to bless us with children.

As we finished praying, a Bible passage filled my mind. It was Psalm

128, which was spoken over us at our send-off prayer party before we left for Houston:

> Blessed are all who fear the LORD, who walk in obedience to him. You will eat the fruit of your labor; blessings and prosperity will be yours. Your wife will be like a fruitful vine within your house; your children will be like olive shoots around your table. Yes, this will be the blessing for the man who fears the LORD. May the LORD bless you from Zion; may you see the prosperity of Jerusalem all the days of your life. May you live to see your children's children—peace be on Israel.

We believed that for our family. We chose to believe that my wife would be a fruitful vine. We trusted that our children would be like olive shoots around our table. We trusted and believed that we would live to see our children's children. That does not mean there wasn't doubt or fear; we just chose as best as we could to believe in that moment. We were like the man in Mark 9 who came to Jesus, desperate for Him to heal his sick son. When Jesus responded by telling him that all things were possible to the one who believes, the man cried, "I do believe; help me overcome my unbelief!" (v. 24).

It is important to note that when we say we "prayed and believed," we still had doubt. We struggled at times to fully believe, especially when doctors' reports were so grim. If you are having trouble believing in something you are praying for, pray this prayer with us: "I do believe; help me overcome my unbelief." Our Father in heaven understands we are human.

We called Aly's mom and the doctor back in and told them we'd decided to start the cancer treatment immediately—the following day, in fact. As much as we wanted a family, Aly and I knew the only way that would ever be possible would be for Aly to live through this ordeal. That was our primary goal. We were choosing to believe that God would protect Aly's womb and that He would completely heal Aly of cancer through the doctors and treatments at MD Anderson. The doctor ran off to put the plan into motion, and we went out to update my parents in the waiting room.

Once again the plan had changed. I couldn't stop thinking, *Can I please get off this roller coaster?*

THE NEW LIFE PLAN

—ALY—

Josh and I used to joke about my life plan; I thought I had everything figured out when we first got married. Boy, was I wrong! I had a new plan now, and it literally was a *life* plan. It was the plan to save my life. That second day at MD Anderson was a wake-up call for me. I realized I had to stop getting knocked around by all the bad news and find my feet again. I'd been a proactive person my whole life; I'm a list maker, a goal setter, and an action-oriented high achiever. Why was I letting cancer push me around now? As heartbreaking as the last few days had been, a new spark started growing inside me. It was the spark to fight back.

After two full days of tests, scans, and consultations, we finally had my cancer treatment protocol: I would undergo sixteen rounds of chemotherapy that would last six months. After chemo, I would have a bilateral mastectomy, which meant removing both of my breasts, followed by thirty rounds of radiation lasting six weeks. Then I'd have a choice whether to have breast reconstruction. If I wanted to do that, I was told to expect a couple more procedures. In all, I was looking at two full years of treatments, surgeries, and recovery time. I wasn't excited about any of it, but my attitude at that point was, *Let's get started.* I certainly wasn't looking forward to cancer treatment, but I *was* looking forward to beating cancer. I wanted it out of my life, and the faster I started, the faster I'd be done with it for good.

During this time we asked the doctors to stop telling us statistics. We found that medical people love throwing stats around, telling you what your chances are for this or that. Josh and I realized that, more often than not, those statistics made us worry even more about what was happening. So we chose not to hear them anymore. I believe a key to getting through any difficulty in life is to fill your mind with things that build your faith. As much as we needed to grasp the seriousness of this situation, we knew that learning the statistics would only bring doubt and fear. Instead, we asked our doctor to tell us in general terms what we needed to know in order to make decisions and to leave "stats for stats' sake" out of our conversations.

Here's what she told us with as few statistics as possible: I was diagnosed with Stage III breast cancer. The cancer was triple negative, meaning it was not grown by the normal three types of hormones typically associated with breast cancer. This type of cancer I had is extremely aggressive and *may or may not* respond to chemotherapy; it was unpredictable. She told us this type of cancer has a high likelihood of recurrence, especially in the first two years after treatment. However, if I made it without recurrence after the first two years, my outcome would probably be very good. And if I made it five years without a recurrence, my outcome should be excellent. This was honestly more detail than we would have liked, but we knew we needed a few specifics to pray about. The two- and five-year milestones became especially big prayer targets for our family.

I'm grateful that God told us early on to avoid unnecessary details that would have worked against our faith. In this day and age, it's so easy to go down internet rabbit holes and dig up every dark, discouraging article about whatever illness we're facing. I know cancer patients who have nearly driven themselves crazy reading every horror story they could find online.

Side note: If all you are reading on the internet are negative stories, realize that oftentimes those are the ones people share. Very seldom do people take the time to tell a success story. I had to remind myself of this often, and that is one of the main reasons I am writing this book. If you're facing a health crisis right now, I encourage you to step away from the computer and give your doctor some guidelines. If too many details are eating away at your faith, it's okay to ask not to hear the details that don't specifically empower you to make decisions. Stay informed, of course, with what you need to know to take care of yourself. Beyond that, immerse yourself in Scripture and other things that will strengthen your faith. Those faith reserves were essential for me during my cancer journey.

LIFE-SAVING POISON

The first step of my cancer fight was chemotherapy. A *lot* of chemotherapy. When we started, the doctor gave me a list of likely side effects. She told me I would probably lose my hair, gain weight, develop acne, have stomach issues, lose my fingernails and toenails, experience numbness in my fingers and toes, and more. Just what every woman wants to hear! It was scary, but we were believing that my side effects would be minimal and that the chemotherapy would go straight to my cancer cells and not damage any healthy cells. It was hard to wrap my head around the fact that to heal my body they had to fill me with poison. How do doctors come up with this stuff?

I assumed I'd spend all day every day in bed once I started chemo, but that's not what happened. After the first treatment, I felt good. *Really* good. It was weird. I also assumed I'd wake up the next morning and find all my hair in a big pile on my pillow, but that didn't happen either. Sure, the side effects came, but it was a gradual process. Thank God! I doubt I'd have handled it very well if everything happened all at once.

I have noticed that oftentimes God builds our character and faith gradually. As badly as I wanted it to all be over, God was having me trust Him for each breath. Had He allowed me to be cancer-free immediately, I would not have the intimacy with Him I now feel or the character that cancer has built in me. Those are not things you buy or can muster up. Sometimes the only way you can experience a certain amount of intimacy with the Lord and build the godly character He desires for us to have is by going through unimaginable pain and gradually, sometimes for years, trusting Him until things get better. The truth that I later learned is that God loved me too much to take my suffering away in the way I wanted Him to. He knew the pain would cause me to draw near to Him and become the person He created me to be. Much easier said in hindsight, let me tell ya!

After the fourth treatment, my hair started coming out whenever I washed or brushed it. I was extremely careful with it at first; I wasn't ready to part with it, so I rarely touched my hair. Any time I did, big clumps would fall out. I had a wig as a backup because I saw the hair loss as a signal to the world that I was sick. When you see a woman who's bald—eyebrows and all—your first thought is that she's a cancer patient, and I didn't want the world to define me as that.

I had to keep reminding myself that the hair loss was a sign the chemo was working. One night, as a clump fell out in front of Josh, he wrapped his arms around me and told me how sorry he was that this was happening. I looked at him and said, "It's okay, baby. That's the cancer falling out!"

—JOSH—

Aly is a fighter, but I knew it was hard for her to face the effects of chemo. The cancer was life-threatening, of course, but it had never made her *feel* sick. That was always tough for me to come to grips with. Aly had no physical symptoms of having cancer, yet she was very, very ill. The chemo, however, was visibly wrecking her body. When she got worried about touching her hair, I volunteered to wash and gently dry it for her. I made a point of always telling her how beautiful she looked—and I meant it.

I'm sure there were times when she heard me say that and thought, *Yeah, right. Despite what they say, bald isn't beautiful.* But it was for her. Spending that time with her, serving her by washing, drying, and brushing her hair, was one of the most precious times of our marriage for me. As her hair came out—first a few strands at a time and then in handfuls—God gave me eyes to see how *truly* beautiful she is. Watching her fight this battle for her life with such faith and grace left me in awe. I thought back to that night when we were teenagers and I saw her reading her Bible in the ski lodge, and once again I asked myself, *Is she out of my league?* Yes, of course she is. But fortunately, she loves me anyway.

—ALY—

Those months of chemotherapy were rough. I lost all my hair, including my eyebrows and eyelashes. My fingernails and toenails turned black and fell off. I had extreme bone pain after rounds of injections. The effects weren't just health-related either. Our lives were crazy for those six months of chemotherapy. We traveled back and forth from Louisiana to Houston every week, but we still fought to retain some sense of normalcy in our lives. We did not want to eat, sleep, and breathe cancer 24-7; we wanted our lives to be about more than my illness. So to the surprise of many people around me, I chose to stick with my PhD program during that time. I was only two months into the degree program when I was diagnosed; I had literally just started. My plan before cancer was to finish my doctorate in three years and start having kids. Well, kids were off the table for a while, but I wasn't ready to give up my goal of finishing my degree in three years. Besides, I had an internship at a counseling clinic already lined up, and I knew my studies would be a great diversion for me.

We stayed so busy during the months of chemo that I didn't give myself much time to sit around and mope about cancer. On Monday, Tuesday, and Wednesday, Josh and I went to work and school. We left for Houston on Thursday, got my treatment on Friday, then headed home to relax a little for the weekend. Then we'd get up Monday morning and start the whole thing again.

Sure, it was crazy for a while, but those were important months for us.

They set the course for our entire cancer journey. I could have spent the whole time in bed, just getting up to go to my chemo treatments, but what kind of life would that have been? Instead, Josh and I chose to believe we'd have a life *after* cancer, and I knew my life after cancer included a PhD and a career in family therapy. So I kept working toward that goal. If I were sitting at home, I might have started to worry or feel sorry for myself, and that was the last thing I needed. While still accepting reality and taking care of myself, I trusted that Jesus had already healed me; I was just waiting to see the manifestation of that miracle.

We kept up that pace for months, right up until my last day of chemotherapy. It was a day to celebrate! Josh woke me up with a video he made for me filled with pictures and videos from my journey. Then we went to the hospital with my family, and my best friends surprised me in Houston for my last treatment. I loved seeing everyone there, but my mind was fixated on the bell mounted on the wall of the cancer center. Every time I went for a checkup or a chemo appointment, I saw that bell. The nurse told me on my first day that I would ring that bell after my last treatment. Today was the day! Praise God!

When that final treatment was over, I got up, walked out to that bell, and rang the heck out of it. We celebrated and screamed and praised God in that room. All the pain, travel, side effects, and prayers were worth it now that I had finished what I was told would be the hardest six months of my cancer battle. What a celebration!

My last ultrasound after chemo took a little of the joy out of the celebration for me, though. I had been praying for months that the chemotherapy would totally eradicate the cancer in my lymph nodes. I believed I had been fully healed of that, but the ultrasound showed otherwise. The doctor took regular ultrasounds throughout my treatment to check on the lymph nodes, and they always showed signs that they were responding to the treatment. The response wasn't always (or even often) dramatic—sometimes there was little or no change—but at least they weren't getting worse. I had really hoped this ultrasound would reveal a miracle, that God had replaced my sick, swollen lymph nodes with perfectly healthy and normal ones.

Well, that didn't happen. The post-chemo ultrasound showed that the lymph nodes were "stable," meaning they still looked abnormal but hadn't gotten worse. The oncologist told me we'd know for sure what was going on with the lymph nodes after they were removed during my mastectomy surgery, but for now, I still had cancer.

NEXT UP: MASTECTOMY

I only had three weeks to catch my breath before it was time to undergo a bilateral mastectomy. To be honest, I wasn't super tied to my breasts. I knew I would be okay without them, though I knew eventually I did want to undergo breast reconstruction. The main thing I was concerned about was how my husband would view me, and I was crushed to know that I couldn't breastfeed if we were able to have children down the road.

As Josh and I waited outside the doctor's office for my mastectomy consult, it dawned on me that he and I had never really talked about what I would look like when all this was over. With the biggest lump in my throat, I finally asked, "Will you still be attracted to me?" It took him a while to respond, which worried me a bit. After sitting in silence for a moment, he said, "Aly, I honestly think I will be *more* attracted to you after the surgery. Every time I look at you, we will be reminded of what Satan tried to do to harm you and how God healed you. That is so very beautiful." Oh, my man. That was the perfect response at the perfect time. It was truly one of the most tender moments we've ever had together.

I think about those words every time I see myself in a mirror. I have visible signs on my body that testify to the healing power of our loving God. Genesis 50:20 inspires me, "You intended to harm me, but God intended it for good to accomplish what is now being done." I have no excuse for ever forgetting what God has done or what He can do in any situation. Do you have something you can put in front of yourself every day to remind you of what God has done in your life? If we're not intentional about reminding ourselves, we'll start to forget—and I never want to forget how faithful God has been in my life.

Of course, I've now had several years to get comfortable with who I am and how I look. Sitting in the doctor's office that day, though, I wondered how Josh could honestly believe that. How could he find me *more* attractive? No hair. No breasts. The guilt I felt for putting him through all this had been piling up. He's the person I love most in the world. The thought of adding so much pain to his life broke my heart. But he wouldn't have it when I started in with my apologies. He told me so many times, "Aly, you haven't done anything to me. Cancer is doing this, and it's doing it to both of us. And we're going to beat it together." So with my amazing husband at my side, we scheduled the mastectomy surgery—the next item on our list.

—JOSH—

Aly had both breasts and nineteen lymph nodes removed on April 23, 2012. It was a long, six-hour surgery, and our friends and family prayed like crazy the entire time. Not only was this a major surgery physically, but it had huge implications for her cancer prognosis. Everything the doctors removed would be tested for cancer, and we would learn if the chemotherapy had worked. That would tell us if Aly was cancer-free or if she'd need further treatment.

After waiting for what seemed like forever, I was finally called back to talk to the doctor and told the surgery was successful and that Aly was doing well. I didn't know what to expect, but I was ready to see her! When I got to her recovery room, Aly was awake and in a tremendous amount of pain. She kept complaining about being hot, so I jumped into action and tried to cool her down. I got ice water and kept putting ice rags all over her. No one was too concerned since she didn't have a fever, but Aly just kept saying how hot she was. In all the years we'd been together, I had *only* known her to be freezing 98 percent of the time. So hearing her complain so much about the room temperature worried me a bit.

The pain and heat continued after she was moved out of recovery and into a regular hospital room. That's when the nausea kicked in too. For the first time in my life, I saw my bride helpless. Even during the worst parts of chemo, Aly had been able to take care of herself, but now she was in excruciating pain, unable to cool off, and throwing up almost nonstop. She had five surgical drains that had to be emptied and recorded. She needed help going to the bathroom. Six months into this journey together, and I think this was the moment that gave us the biggest reality check about what our lives would look like for the foreseeable future.

Aly was able to get more comfortable and cool off when we finally got her home, but she still needed around-the-clock care. I also knew at some point she would need help removing her bandages and cleaning the surgical site. Neither of us discussed how we'd handle that; I just waited for her lead. I had been preparing my heart and mind for this moment, though. I knew my reaction would be *everything* to her and that it would be a moment neither of us would ever forget.

The day finally arrived when Aly asked me to help her remove the bandages. She said she was ready for both of us to see her scars (she hadn't seen herself yet either). As I carefully undid the bandages, I didn't cry or freak out in any way. I was honestly surprised about how calm I was. I peeled away the last bandage and stepped back to look at my wife. She was stunning. That's the only word I can use to describe how she looked: *stunning*. There she was, my beautiful Aly, with a completely flat chest and two scars. I told her how beautiful she was, kissed those two perfect scars, and turned her to face the mirror with me at her side. With all the horrors we'd been through, this was one of the most beautiful moments of our lives. I couldn't imagine loving her more than I did in that moment.

CHAPTER 4

BROKEN AND HEALED

—ALY—

I spent the week after my mastectomy recovering at home. Those first few days were harder than I'd expected they would be. The hot flashes were driving me crazy, and the nausea was out of control. That was the sickest I'd ever felt. Add to that the emotional impact of losing my breasts, worrying about what Josh would think of me when he saw my new body, and the uncertainty of whether the surgery removed all the cancer, and let's just say it wasn't the best week for me.

Josh was amazing, though. He was right there with me through all of it, doing whatever he could to make me comfortable. And of course I will never forget the moment he took off my bandages. I knew Josh loved me, and we'd been through a lot together. But that experience took things to a whole other level. I had never felt more loved than I did right then.

My follow-up appointment was scheduled for one week post-op, on April 30. That was a huge appointment. That's when the doctors would tell us if the chemotherapy had been successful. After they removed all of my breast tissue and lymph nodes, they would biopsy it all to see if the chemo-therapy had killed the cancer cells. Many people have surgery first and then chemotherapy, but my process was the opposite. Most may never know if the chemotherapy really did its job because they have the cancer removed in surgery and then do chemotherapy. Since I was doing chemotherapy first, I was about to have tangible evidence of whether the cancer was shrinking in response to the treatment.

I spent that week praying and believing that God had healed me. I forced every speck of doubt out of my mind and fully trusted in God's healing power. I was excited for my upcoming doctor's appointment because I knew—I just *knew*—that my cancer nightmare was coming to a close. As Josh and I talked about the future, though, I realized he and I weren't totally on the same page.

As I talked about getting an "all clear" report from the doctor, Josh kept dropping in what-if comments. What if I wasn't completely cancer-free? What if I needed more treatments? He talked about where we could stay in Houston for an extended period of time if we needed to. He wondered what he could do about his job if we had to keep driving back and forth to Houston. None of this was *bad* in and of itself. I get that, as my husband, he was focused on taking care of me and supporting our family no matter what came our way. He'd been an incredible partner throughout this whole journey; I couldn't imagine going through everything that had happened without him at my side. However, every what-if he mentioned felt like bamboo under my fingernails (well, that's how it would have felt if I still *had* fingernails back then). As we looked toward my April 30 appointment, I realized I had to reset some expectations.

"Josh, I need you to believe. I need you to stop making backup plans and simply *believe* with me that I'm healed of this cancer." He was startled—probably because I was visibly irritated with him and my tone confirmed it.

We've had hundreds of important conversations throughout our relationship. Sometimes we both get super engaged and argue back and forth. Sometimes one of us will drop a truth bomb and the other one will immediately *get it* and apologize or agree. I was prepared for either of those scenarios, but this was something different. Josh just sat there silently. I could tell he was really thinking about what I'd said. Neither of us said much else the rest of the night. We simply held hands in bed and drifted off to sleep. I prayed for him intensely in that silence. I needed him to believe—I needed us *both* to believe—that I was healed.

The next morning I could tell a change had happened in Josh. I believe the Holy Spirit was at work in him, settling his fears and bringing us together in full faith. From that point on, Josh started talking about April 30 as a good day, a day of celebration. He commented on how wonderful it would be to get the good news from the doctor that my cancer was gone. He didn't say a word about any backup plans. I was amazed at how much his renewed faith strengthened my own.

God taught us both a powerful lesson that night. If someone is doing or saying things that weaken your faith—even if it's a spouse, friend, or mentor—be courageous enough to tell them to set aside their doubts and believe with you. Jesus calls us to be bold in our belief, reminding us, "I will do whatever you ask in my name, so that the Father may be glorified in the Son. You may ask me for anything in my name, and I will do it" (John 14:13–14). It's hard to maintain that level of faith when the people closest to us are dragging us down, so be careful in your relationships. Ask the people you love to join you in believing, and if there are others around who just won't stop speaking negativity into your life, tell them to stop. You might even need to walk away from some relationships for a while. That's okay! Be kind, but be faithful to the belief God has put in your heart.

FAITH MANIFESTED

The day finally arrived. Even though I was believing for a clear report from the doctor, I couldn't help but think back to a conversation we'd had with the oncologist before my mastectomy. As much as we tried to avoid hearing statistics throughout my treatment, one would occasionally slip past our defenses. That had been one of those times. She wanted to be sure we understood that my chances of being cancer-free after the mastectomy were less than 20 percent.

Dang! That's exactly the type of stat we tried to avoid. But throughout the surgery and the week after, that number kept popping into my head. Yes, I *believed* I was cancer-free, but occasionally I'd hear an inner voice of doubt say, *But there's an 80 percent chance you're not.* Man, statistics are terrible.

So as we walked into the oncologist's office on April 30, 2012, the words "less than 20 percent" kept screaming in my head. Then I'd heard a little whisper in my spirit that said, "By My stripes you are healed," echoing Isaiah 53:5 (NKJV). Isn't it funny that the negative voices seem so much louder than the others? It takes faith and conscious effort to push those voices aside so we can focus on the still, small voice of the Spirit. If we have accepted Christ into our hearts, we can trust that we have His Spirit within us—even when fear and doubt try to drown out His voice.

Josh and I sat nervously waiting in the doctor's office. Hey, faith doesn't mean the nerves don't get the best of us every now and then, right? When the doctor finally walked in, a second doctor trailed in behind her. In my experience, seeing *two* doctors when you expected *one* had never meant good news. I squeezed Josh's hand and took a breath.

The doctor said, "Hey, guys, this is Dr. Somethingorother." Yeah, I forgot his name as soon as she said it. She continued, "I always like to have another doctor with me when I deliver good news."

"It's . . . it's *good* news?" we asked. Was this really about to happen?

"No, it's not *good* news; it's *perfect* news!" She continued, "This almost never happens so soon after a mastectomy, but I can tell you that you are completely cancer-free!" She explained that the lymph nodes still looked cancerous on the ultrasound, but all the breast tissue and lymph nodes came back totally clear with no evidence of disease anywhere.

Cue the sobbing! And shouting! And praise dancing! Seriously, *praise dancing*. The oncologist told us the other doctor she brought in was the pharmacist who prescribed my chemotherapy regimen, and they both agreed that I needed no further treatment except to complete my radiation as planned. I was cancer-free. CANCER-FREE! After spending days and weeks and months being poked and prodded nonstop by a million different doctors, the oncologist told me she didn't need to see me again for three months. And just like that, I was kicked out of cancer treatment—*because I didn't have cancer anymore!* Josh and I fell into each other's arms sobbing and praising God for healing me. We walked out of that office on cloud nine. It was the first truly good day we'd had since the whole ordeal began, and we wanted to feel every ounce of joy we could squeeze out of the experience.

As Josh and I were leaving the oncologist's office, a woman approached me as she had been following my blog online. It was like I was a celebrity! She had been diagnosed with triple negative breast cancer while she was pregnant. With tears in her eyes, she was able to tell me how much my blog impacted her and gave her inspiration. Once again I was learning how important it had been to share my story online. What she didn't know was the news I had just received. I was able to give her the biggest hug and tell her she was the first person to hear I was cancer-free! Her whole face lit up, and she told us how grateful she was to hear our story. Knowing that miracles do happen, that God truly does heal His people, meant the world to her in that moment. I believe God put that woman in front of me at the perfect time to remind me to never stop sharing my story, and to shout it from the rooftops if necessary.

When God works a miracle in our lives, we have a duty to share it with those around us. It truly may mean the difference between life and death for those still struggling. Looking back on April 30, 2012, I'm not only thankful for the incredible news I got from the doctor; I'm also grateful for that immediate opportunity to give someone hope by speaking of God's healing power. He had given me the words of life, and in His name, my life was saved. "LORD my God, I called out to you for help, and you healed me" (Psalm 30:2). He really did it! Praise God!

CANCER'S SUCKER PUNCH

—JOSH—

I can't even begin to describe how I felt when I got that doctor's report. We had desperately prayed for good news at every step of this journey, but it seemed like every doctor's appointment only took us deeper down the cancer pit. But now my wife was cancer-free.

I would love to say our cancer battle ended for good after that doctor's appointment, but Aly's fight wasn't quite over yet. There were still two big hurdles in front of us. As Aly said, she still had to go through six weeks of radiation as planned. And there was also the matter of her breast reconstruction. Little did we know that two months of intense radiation would be the *easy* part!

We had about a month "off" from worrying about surgeries, tests, treatments, and commutes to Houston before Aly had to report for radiation. This phase of treatment would take two months, so we relocated to Houston for the summer of 2012. Cyd had friends from college, Lance and Tammy Stanfill, who live in Houston, and they became what we refer to as our "Houston family." We lived with them during that summer, and that was one of the most unforgettable summers of our lives for many reasons. Even though we had been through nearly six months of chemotherapy and I knew how horrible cancer treatment could be, I was still surprised by what I saw during Aly's radiation treatment. The burns on her skin were awful. She looked like she had third-degree burns all over her chest. I had the same thought I'd had so often during chemo: *How is this supposed to help her?*

As her husband and champion, it was hard for me to sit by and watch her go off to essentially experience torture. Aly, however, was amazing. She was her typical "get it done" self and rallied through every treatment, no matter how much it hurt. She demonstrated the most beautiful, rock-solid faith the whole time. She had believed for a healing miracle, and God had given it to her. If putting up with a summer of radiation treatments was part of the deal, she was willing do it.

We still managed to have some fun that summer, though. The Stanfills are forever a part of our family, and we can never thank them enough for opening their home to us. We also welcomed visitors as our friends and family came to spend time with us in Houston, and Aly and I spent a ton of time together talking about life and getting a vision for what our cancer-free future would look like. She still had several more surgeries before then, though.

After radiation came reconstruction, and that *did not* go well. She was rushed in for two different emergency surgeries following her main reconstruction procedure, and all this trauma took a toll on my wife. As much as she likes to take charge and attack problems head-on, the reconstruction phase brought her to the point of complete helplessness again. (Aly will talk more about these surgeries and complications later in the book.) I honestly didn't realize how painful this part of the process would be for her. Neither of us did. We simply were not expecting such hard times to continue after she was declared cancer-free. We thought we were almost off this roller-coaster ride when the oncologist gave us the good news, but the reconstruction surgeries took more out of Aly than anything else we had experienced.

After one of these surgeries, Aly really needed a shower. She felt gross, and she knew she would feel better after washing off. However, she couldn't walk, lift her arms, or do much of anything other than lie in bed. So a nurse had to come in and bathe her. I tried to help as much as I could, but I will never forget Aly being so helpless while a nurse washed her. I knew Aly was mortified, and once again we had to keep our eyes on the goal: a healthy life that shines the light of Christ.

We prayed that these hardships would bring the perseverance promised in Scripture. Remembering the night Aly told me flatly that she needed me to believe with her, I was dead set on focusing on her complete recovery. I realized that it is one thing to read and believe the Bible in a vacuum, but it's an entirely different level of faith to believe God's Word of healing when you're watching a nurse bathe your weak, helpless, and weeping wife.

JOSH'S CANCER TREATMENT

Watching Aly—the love of my life—go through such horrors and being completely unable to help her or take the burden from her destroyed me on many levels. While she felt helpless to do things for herself, I felt . . . powerless. This was devastating to me as a man. As she fought for her life, I started to realize that her cancer treatment was changing *me* as well as changing her. It was forcing me to take a good, hard look at myself and the faith I clung to. Now, looking back over the past seven-plus years since her initial diagnosis, I can say without a doubt that today I am a much different man. God and cancer changed me through and through, and that transformation really came into focus as I watched the nurse bathe Aly.

There were a handful of moments throughout our journey that seemed surreal, and watching a total stranger wash my wife's body seemed like the ultimate violation of personal space. It was a powerful reminder that, as active as we'd been in attacking her cancer, none of this was in our control. This wasn't just *pain*. This was the pinnacle of humiliation and helplessness. More than that, I came to realize this was a picture of our complete surrender to God—only I hadn't surrendered everything to Him yet.

I said cancer had changed me, but I hadn't allowed *God* to fully change me yet. I was still trying to control things, primarily our finances. Even as Aly struggled to recover from her surgeries, I was nursing new business ideas and financial opportunities. I was worried about jobs, paychecks, and medical bills. There was no doubt God was telling me to stay in the job I was in and to spend every other ounce of energy caring for and spending time with Aly. He had big plans for our family; only He knew what awaited us on the other side of cancer. I believe He wanted me focused on Aly and our marriage in these critical years, fighting not only for Aly's life but also for our future together. And yet I kept chasing after other things in my mind, chasing rabbits I know weren't from God. I realized God had given me the ability to lead Aly through this; I just wasn't giving Him the ability to lead *me*.

God broke me through Aly's cancer. He broke my self-reliance. He broke my preoccupation with finances. He broke the plans I had set for myself and my family. And then He stepped into that brokenness and started showing me what *He* had planned for us. I didn't know exactly what the future held for us, what the rest of Aly's fight would be like, whether we'd be able to have children, or what our careers would look like. But I did know He was already there, shaping and holding our future in His hands—the same hands that had healed my wife of life-threatening cancer. If I could trust my wife's life to those nail-scarred hands, I knew I could trust our finances to them too.

I wish I could say this was an overnight change for me, bringing me new faith and confidence like a light in the darkness. But it wasn't. It was a start, though. God had broken me, picked up the pieces, and started building something new. And I knew He would finish His work in His time.

—ALY—

Watching the transformation happen in my husband was truly incredible. People come up to me all the time and say, "I knew Josh in high school, and he was a nice guy," or "Josh used to coach my son in basketball. He was great."

Almost every time I'll say something like, "Yeah, he was pretty great back then—but you should meet him *now*! He's a completely different person." Seeing what God has done in and through him has been an unexpected blessing of my cancer.

Since then, brokenness has been a common topic for us, especially for Josh. He's become passionate about sharing his story of brokenness to others and explaining how God has built an amazing, unexpected new life from the shattered pieces.

One night as we were lying in bed, Josh was going on and on in one of his many minisermons about brokenness when I stopped him mid-sentence and said, "Josh, do you realize you are *healed*? I know you were broken before God and you continue to be broken, but do you know you are also healed?" Once again he responded to my gentle rebuke with silence. I could tell I had spun his mind off in a different direction, and I was curious where it would go.

—JOSH—

Aly has a way of hitting me in the gut with truth. She was right. I had spent so much time focused on my brokenness that I hadn't paid much attention to the fact that God had healed me. Yes, God had broken me, and I rejoiced in that. He broke me of some patterns and thoughts that would have led me far away from where He wanted me to be. But Aly was showing me that God didn't *leave* me broken. He took those shattered pieces of who I was and used them to make me into a new creation in Christ. From that point on, I kept telling people about the power of brokenness, but I also emphasized how that's only half the conversation. The other side of the coin is the healing that comes after the brokenness. That's the real power—the ongoing daily cycle of brokenness and healing. I believe that's how God continually molds and refines us into the men and women He's called us to be. That's the message I now spread every chance I get. That's what God taught me during *my* cancer treatment.

CHAPTER 5

CANCER'S AFTERMATH

—ALY—

I talked to many cancer survivors while I was fighting my battle, and I was shocked to hear them say that one of the hardest parts of the whole journey for them was getting back to life *after* cancer. Like I said in the previous chapter, I always thought life would go back to normal at that point. I remember thinking, *What in the world are they talking about? When I'm cancer-free, I'll shout from the rooftops! It'll be the best time of my life!* I believed that with my whole heart, but once I got there myself, I quickly understood cancer's aftermath and what it can do to you if you don't keep up your guard.

When my doctor told me I was cancer-free, she basically discharged me. I was prepared to keep coming back for regular checkups, but she only needed to see me every three months. Otherwise, she said to call with any questions or concerns. Before she let me go, however, she made sure I understood that my type of cancer had a high likelihood of recurrence, especially within the first two years. So she stressed to me how important it was to let her know if anything felt . . . *odd*. I had no idea how much that statement would affect my life over the following years.

As we left the hospital that day, I was on cloud nine. I was alive! I was going to live! Life was going to be (somewhat) normal again! It's one thing to believe you will be healed, as I'd done throughout the whole ordeal. It was something else entirely to see it actually come to pass. Thank You, Jesus!

—JOSH—

As we left that day, my biggest thought was, *Well, what do we do now?* We'd been prepared for more treatments and another phase of cancer life, but instead, the journey just *stopped.* Aly was cancer-free. Everything we'd been praying for and believing for had come to pass. What now?

When we were living with cancer, we did everything we could to make life feel *normal.* But it wasn't normal. At all. Cancer changes everything. It wrecks your plans and dreams. It causes crazy emotions and stretches your faith in all directions. Looking back, it was kind of silly for us to expect our life to snap back to what we once considered normal after Aly got the all clear from her doctor. Plus, with the benefit of time, we're now grateful that God allowed our plans to be wrecked because He had something so much better in store for us. We couldn't see that at the time, though. In that moment, trying to adjust to life after cancer was harder than we ever dreamed.

NEXT STOP: MORE SURGERIES

—ALY—

The next stop after completing all my cancer treatment was reconstructive surgery. We've already mentioned that this process did not go well. The surgeries were eventually successful, but I had issues with my tissue expanders, the devices put under the chest muscle to prepare for the implants that would be placed later. Those issues led me into several emergency surgeries that kept me in near-constant pain for nine months. Everything hurt. My chest. My arms. My back. The pain and swelling were worse when lying flat, and I couldn't even think about lying on my stomach, which was my favorite way to sleep premastectomy, and I had to sleep sitting up for several months.

All that pain and trouble took a terrible toll on me. I remember the doctors reassuring me that I would be glad I was doing this reconstructive phase, but I had moments when I didn't care if I had a flat chest forever; I just wanted to stop hurting and feel normal.

It didn't help that I was in my midtwenties. It was the period of my life when all my friends were getting married, having children, and experiencing their happiest moments. But I was stuck in bed, propped up on a million pillows and emptying surgical drains every hour. I was so tired. Tired of the pain and surgeries. Tired of trying to sleep sitting up. Tired of not being able to sleep on my stomach, which I hadn't done in a year. Tired of not being able to cuddle with my husband. Tired of being a patient.

Finally, nearly a year after I'd been declared cancer-free, all the reconstructive surgeries were over. However, things still weren't *normal* the way we had hoped. Despite the great work of my doctors, my breasts looked much different than they did before cancer and my mastectomy. I was told they'd look somewhat normal when all was said and done, but they weren't normal *for me*. Because so much tissue had been removed during my mastectomy, there wasn't enough left to support my previous breast size. As a result, the doctors had to make my reconstructed breasts much smaller than they were originally.

So not only did I have to get used to implants, but I also had to get used to the fact that I looked so different. I wondered if I would ever feel like myself again, and if I didn't, how would I deal with that? I didn't really know the answer. I had to trust God with each step. What I *did* know was that I was cancer-free and there were no more surgeries in my future. We felt like we had finally climbed over a huge hump and that life was going to calm down a little bit.

IS THE CANCER BACK?

—JOSH—

We were so relieved when Aly's surgeries were over. After a nonstop roller-coaster ride for the past year and a half, we were ready for a break. Before we could really relax, though, Aly started having new pain. It started in her leg and hips. The doctor had warned us to pay attention to anything that felt off, so we weren't sure what to think of these new symptoms. Aly had been in so much pain for so long, it became hard to figure out what pain was new and what was old. This was different, though.

She started complaining to me about hip and back pain, and I had to be extremely careful in my reactions. I knew from experience that if I seemed overly concerned, Aly could start freaking out. But if I didn't seem concerned *enough*, Aly might think I didn't believe she was really having these symptoms.

The doctor's warning kept ringing in our ears, so we filtered every ache and pain through the lens of, *Is this the cancer coming back?* We made a decision not to live in fear, but that is easier said than done when Aly was supposed to be highly sensitive to any new pain, and she was having many new pains! It really messed with our minds in ways we weren't expecting. It's like we got off one horrible ride and climbed right back onto another. We were not prepared for the aftermath of cancer at all.

—ALY—

It was so hard not to believe that the cancer had come back in a different part of my body. I clung to Nahum 1:9: "Affliction shall not rise up the second time" (KJV). While I believed this and trusted that God had healed me, I knew others whose cancer had returned. That made it difficult for me to fully believe, but I kept fighting for my faith. As always, I prayed, "I do believe; help me overcome my unbelief!" (Mark 9:24). During these two weeks of struggling with this new hip and back pain, I felt like I was having to settle a key question in my spirit once and for all: *Am I scared of cancer?* As I was crying to a friend about this, she said (pretty frankly), "Aly, you can't be scared of cancer. God is bigger than cancer." I know that may sound like a simple statement, but it made me realize how much fear I'd allowed cancer to cram into my life. I didn't want to be a person of fear; I'm a person of *faith*!

I spent so much time during this ordeal reading the psalms. Having fought this battle for so long, I felt a close connection to David as he continually cried out to God. He always seemed to be in trouble, facing insurmountable odds and desperately in need of rescue. One of my favorite passages during this time was Psalm 3:

> Lord, how many are my foes! How many rise up against me! Many are saying of me, "God will not deliver him." But you, Lord, are a shield around me, my glory, the One who lifts my head high. I call out to the Lord, and he answers me from his holy mountain. I lie down and sleep; I wake again, because the Lord sustains me. I will not fear though tens of thousands assail me on every side. Arise, Lord! Deliver me, my God! Strike all my enemies on the jaw; break the teeth of the wicked. From the Lord comes deliverance. May your blessing be on your people.

Like David, there were times when I felt my enemy, cancer, "assail me on every side." Even though I was cancer-free, the shadow of cancer was always present, often making us worry and second-guess everything I felt in my body. I never lost faith that God had healed me . . . but some days it was hard to hold on to that faith.

The hip and back pain eventually took us back to Houston for a checkup with my doctor and a bone scan. Thankfully, the scan was clear, but we did discover a bulging disc in my back. It wasn't cancer-related—yay!—but you can see how exhausting it was to always have to ask the question, "Is this a cancer symptom?" That's a question that became even more real to me when I got a heartbreaking piece of news during my back ordeal.

Early in my cancer journey, I got to know two women who had walked the road of breast cancer before me—Donna and Amy. Their diagnoses weren't as dire as mine, but it meant the world to me for them to reach out and offer their guidance. They gave me advice on shaving my head, came over to my house to show me their mastectomy scars, and talked me through the ups and downs of reconstruction. These ladies were also great sounding boards for all the fears I had about cancer.

As my back pain first became an issue, I got the heart-wrenching news that Donna had a breast cancer recurrence. I wish I could say that I rallied around her and supported her, but I didn't. Fear entrenched me. I was so scared for her—and scared for me. *Would this same thing happen to me? Why is this happening to her?* I didn't understand. I don't understand cancer at all—why some people are healed and why some people aren't. I know we live in a fallen world full of illness and disease, but still . . . watching people you love go through the hell of cancer is something you can't put into words.

My friend passed away a few months later. I couldn't bring myself to go to the funeral; it was just too hard. I honestly thought I might pass out, or at the very least cry uncontrollably if I were there. My heart broke for my friend and the husband and daughter she left behind. She had been such a shining light for me, and now she was gone. I was mourning and angry. And scared. Scared that this could happen to me too. It was too much for my heart and mind to bear at times.

PARALYZING FEAR

Eventually, after a few months of physical therapy, my back got better. I had to keep reminding myself that my body had been through the wringer, and I was probably going to have a lot of aches and pains for a while as a result of all the surgeries and treatments. But dealing with these new pains while managing my fear of a recurrence *and* mourning the loss of a survivor sister . . . this wasn't exactly the *normal* life I thought I'd go back to after cancer. Josh and I started to realize that survivorship could be a rough road.

Then, as my back finally stopped hurting, a new symptom jumped up and kicked me in the gut—quite literally. I began having severe stomach pain, and it hurt all the time. I complained to Josh about it nonstop, and he did his best to try to calm me down. He'd say it wasn't cancer, he'd pray for me, and he encouraged me to get it checked out. But I was *so tired* of going to doctors. Was I supposed to go to a doctor for every pain? Doctors and doctors' offices had become such a huge source of anxiety for me. I couldn't bear the thought of spending one more minute in a doctor's office. But *not going* freaked me out just as much, because it made me worry that the cancer was growing inside my body again.

It was like a war was being waged between my body and my spirit, and I didn't know what to do anymore. I was afraid that going to the doctor at the drop of a hat meant that my faith was weak, that I didn't *really* believe in the healing God had given me. That may seem silly, but it became a huge obstacle for me. How could I trust in God's healing *and* run off to the doctor for every ache?

I ultimately decided to get my stomach checked out. While we were waiting for the results of my colonoscopy and endoscopy, I was secretly crumbling inside. I have no doubt that Satan was attacking me pretty hard that week. I couldn't find any rest. When I was awake, I was scared of a cancer recurrence. When I went to sleep, I was assaulted by the most horrible nightmares you can imagine. I would never say it out loud, but I was terrified the cancer had returned. As the fear grew greater, I tried to speak words of greater faith. I believed Proverbs 18:21: "The tongue has the power of life and death, and those who love it will eat its fruit." This conflict between my faith and my fear was driving me crazy!

The colonoscopy came back clear, and the doctor said everything looked fine. It was still hard for me to believe that, though. The pain was so intense, I was convinced there was something wrong with me. A few people suggested that it might be anxiety-related, but I dismissed the idea. I think I had always thought of anxiety as *imaginary* pain. The pain I was having, though, was real. I wasn't making it up. So I scheduled a CT scan to get to the bottom of it. I prayed through the entire scan, singing praise songs with tears streaming down my face. I kept saying over and over again, "Please heal me, Jesus. I know I'm healed. Please keep me well."

Two days later, a nurse called with the results. "Mrs. Taylor," she said, "the results showed nothing abnormal." I fell to my knees on our living room floor, shouting and crying, praising God for this news. We had done every test possible to make sure nothing was wrong with my stomach, and we now knew for sure that it wasn't cancer. Yes, it hurt like crazy, but it wasn't cancer!

I rejoiced, but I also prayed more than ever for some relief. Relief from all the pains and fear. Relief from all the symptoms that may or may not be signs that cancer was returning. I was tied up in knots. Looking back, I realize my stomach pain was most likely due to anxiety. I had been through so much with my cancer, I had just lost my friend to her cancer recurrence, and—let's not forget—I was *still* working on my PhD through all this. I was drowning and didn't realize how much I was letting the pressure build up.

I'm a little embarrassed that I didn't even consider anxiety as a cause of the stomach pain. I *am* a therapist, after all. I know how serious anxiety is and how powerful its affects are on the body. But before that experience, I'm ashamed to say I thought patients often exaggerated their symptoms. Boy, was I wrong. As much as it hurt, I'm glad I got that new perspective on anxiety. It's real, and it causes *real* pain. And sadly, I was about to learn how bad depression can be too.

DOWNWARD SPIRAL

—JOSH—

Figuring out what life was supposed to be after cancer was rough. I felt like I should have been the most grateful person on earth, but it was more frustrating than anything. We were lonely. We felt as though our lives had been on pause while everyone else had moved on. Aly and I had spent so much time in Houston, huddled together fighting this battle, that our friends had developed tighter bonds with each other—bonds we weren't a part of. I'm not saying they did anything wrong; they absolutely didn't. Those things just happen when you are away for as long as we were. Our friends were great friends to us when we needed them, but they had their own lives. Even our main cancer mentors, Richard and Angie—the godly couple we mentioned earlier who had become such a big part of our lives—were at a different stage of life. They were older and had teenagers and a full life. It was hard for Aly and me to find our place among all these new dynamics when we got back.

It was a continual battle for me to stay focused on my work. I had been nursing other business ideas, but I felt strongly that God was telling me to set those aside and only focus on Aly and on my school job during that part of our journey. There were times, though, when I longed for an escape. It would have been so easy for me to get lost in a new real estate deal or some other business opportunity. As much as I loved my wife and wanted to be there for her every step of the way, it was hard to see her in pain all the time and to hear this nonstop flood of fear and worry. I wanted so badly for life to be normal, but neither of us even knew what that meant anymore. Every time we got past one hurdle, we ran headlong into the next. First it was the cancer, then the reconstruction, then the back pain, then the stomach pain. Next stop: debilitating headaches.

—ALY—

First Peter 5:8 warns, "Be alert and of sober mind. Your enemy the devil prowls around like a roaring lion looking for someone to devour." For a while, it seemed like the devil only had eyes for me. We kept getting hit by one thing after another, and the enemy kept attacking the things I feared most. After my stomach pain got under control, I started getting headaches. But these weren't normal headaches; the pain was excruciating, like nothing I'd ever experienced before. My entire head hurt from front to back, side to side, and inside out. I'd had headaches before, but nothing like this. Of course I was scared. This was new, and I knew what I was supposed to do when I experienced a new, troublesome symptom. But I couldn't mention it to Josh or anyone else at first. I was so tired of having "symptoms." I desperately wanted to be able to honestly answer, "I feel great!" whenever someone asked me how I was doing. But that day never seemed to come.

I told Josh about the headaches after a few days of suffering alone, and we started the rounds to figure out what it was. I took medicine. I went to an acupuncturist. I went to the chiropractor. I got several head and neck massages. I considered getting shots. Once again I was in continual, nonstop pain. I was *done*.

All the physical torment of the past couple of years finally took its emotional toll on me, and I fell into a deep depression. I was in so much pain I didn't want to get out of bed. Then I would feel guilty that I didn't want to get out of bed. I would tell myself, "I'm healed of cancer! Why would I not want to get out of bed and celebrate every day?" But then I'd get a flash of fear that the headaches were a sign of the cancer returning, and I'd spin off into a deeper depression. It was a horrific cycle, and I could tell Josh was caught up in it too. We'd been trying to "go about life like normal" (funny that we were *still* using this phrase), but we weren't paying attention to the growing threat right in front of our faces.

I needed help. I knew I was in a dark place. I had always been a very positive person, always seeing the glass half full. Not anymore. All the glasses were empty. I saw only two options before me: I either had cancer again, or I was going to live in excruciating pain for the rest of my life. Having been trained in depression and suicidal ideation, I knew I had to talk to someone.

One night I got out of bed and walked into the living room where Josh was sitting. I tried to explain my pain to him and how I felt like I was suffocating. Suffocating from fear and pain and not wanting to live. He stopped me and repeated, "Not wanting to live?"

With tears streaming down my face and my voice quivering, I answered, "Yes. I cannot live like this. I don't *want* to live like this." I told him I didn't have a suicide plan, but I was in a very dark place. Let me tell you, I never, *never* thought those words would come out of my mouth. I was the positive, cheerful, action-oriented, goal-minded woman, remember? I could do anything I set my mind to! But I couldn't do *this*. Not anymore. It was a stark reminder that we are all vulnerable, and we must all stay on guard against the enemy's schemes. He wants to devour us, and he will—if we give him the chance.

Josh looked like he'd seen a ghost. He never expected to hear those words come out of my mouth, but there they were. He immediately called Angie and Richard. I didn't hear what he told them, but he apparently let them know it was urgent, because we headed straight to their house.

As we sat there with them, they asked how we were doing. I just sobbed and sobbed. I couldn't stop crying. I told them of my head pain. I told them I didn't want to do this anymore. Then Richard asked a question that is forever engrained in my mind. He said, "Aly, what is your biggest fear?" I took a minute to think and compose myself a little.

"Dying," I said. "Getting cancer again and my family watching me die."

There was just silence. I honestly don't remember what anyone said after that, but there was freedom in simply saying my fears out loud. No one had ever asked me that, and I guess it was something that was always on my mind. It was an awful lot to carry; I felt lighter just getting it out. After processing and praying with Angie and Richard, I assured them I was not going to take my life, and Josh and I went back home.

Angie and Richard did encourage me to get a brain scan to find out what was going on. Another test, another scan. Ugh . . .

—JOSH—

When we got home that night, I felt a tremendous responsibility to pray over Aly. Sure, I was dealing with a lot of emotions myself, but my wife was considering ending her life? What in the world? I knew I had to take action, and it was a reality check for me about how much Aly was struggling. She needed me more than I could have imagined. I felt led by God to anoint her with oil, so I got some olive oil from the kitchen (it's okay to laugh) and prayed over her like I'd never prayed before. James 5:14 says, "Is anyone among you sick? Let them call the elders of the church to pray over them and anoint them with oil in the name of the Lord." I'm not a church elder, but God had appointed me the spiritual leader of our home, and it was time for me to step up. I confessed Jesus's blood over her life, and we rebuked Satan and told him he had no power over our lives. We recognized we were in a spiritual battle, and we knew we already had the victory in Jesus Christ.

We went to sleep that night exhausted from a long day of pain, honest (but frightening) discussions, eye-opening revelations, and spiritual warfare. All we could do was pray for Aly's brain scan and continue to believe the healing that Jesus had brought about in her.

—ALY—

Before long, I was back in the hospital for a brain CT scan. Every time I'd had any type of scan before then, I'd spent the whole time praying or singing songs, trusting God for the results. By now, though, I had no words left to pray. My mind was blank. I knew I'd go crazy if I didn't do *something* to keep my mind busy during the scan, so I did something I'd never done in any of the dozens of tests and scans I'd been through before. I simply said the name of Jesus over and over. My mother-in-law had recently suggested that, when I didn't know what else to pray, His name was enough. His name is all-powerful, far more powerful than any prayer my human mind could string together. More powerful than any song I could sing or scripture I could recite. His name, the name of Jesus, is enough. So over and over, throughout the entire scan, I repeated His name in my head and out loud. "Jesus, Jesus, Jesus, Jesus."

The first part of the MRI lasted about twenty minutes. Then they pulled me out to inject the contrast dye for the second half of the scan. As the technician inserted my IV for the contrast dye, he looked at me with a smile and said, "You can relax." I've heard that from a lot of lab techs, so I tried to relax as much as I could with a giant plastic thing stuck to my head and half my body still jammed inside an MRI tube. Then he touched me and said again, this time a little more forcefully, "Aly. You can *relax* . . . if you know what I mean." It dawned on me what he was trying to communicate. He was telling me, even though he technically wasn't supposed to, that he didn't see anything to worry about on the scan. I lost it. Tears poured down my face, but I couldn't move my arms in the tube to wipe them off. I finished the scan praising God for reminding me who I am. I proclaimed in that little metal tube, "I am Aly Taylor, child of God, and I am cancer-free!"

The doctor followed up afterward to let me know that the scan was indeed clear. No obvious problem in my brain. No cancer! That was such a relief, but the headaches continued—until they vanished. For six whole months—from April through October 2013—I had a debilitating headache *every single day*. One amazing October morning I woke up and my headaches were gone. Completely gone, and they never came back. Praise God! There is truly power in the name, the simple, all-powerful, healing name of Jesus Christ! I just had to hold on long enough.

If you are still waiting for your breakthrough, keep holding on. Keep walking in faith. And when you can't find the words, say His name. Jesus. Call on Him. He is there.

—JOSH—

It was such a relief for us when Aly's headaches disappeared. Finally—*finally*—things seemed to be looking up. For the first time in two years, my wife was able to get up and face the day without pain. You can't understand how that feels unless you've lived it.

We were also coming up on the two-year anniversary of Aly's cancer diagnosis, a key milestone in cancer recovery where the chance of recurrence drops significantly. Slowly but surely, the darkness started to lift, and we began to see the sun peeking through the clouds again.

Those days of recovery weren't without pain of their own, though. You'll remember that Aly had two key cancer survivors, Donna and Amy, who reached out to her during her treatment. Donna had recently passed away from a recurrence. And as Aly recovered from her headache episodes, I got word that her surviving friend, Amy, had also been diagnosed with a recurrence. I had to call Aly and tell her on the phone, and the news was met by silence on the other end. I knew she was glad I told her, but she was so heartbroken, confused, and scared for her friend. And maybe scared for her own life again too. We hate cancer so much.

CANCER PTSD

—ALY—

As a therapist I have worked with many people who were formally diagnosed with post-traumatic stress disorder (PTSD). It's usually associated with people who have returned from war or have survived similarly traumatic events or abuse. As I went through the painful daily struggle of cancer's aftermath, I realized that PTSD is a real and present danger for cancer survivors as well. If I smelled a certain smell, heard a certain sound, or felt a familiar pain (or *unfamiliar* pain, for that matter), I would get this feeling of panic and fear. Or when I heard of someone getting a cancer diagnosis for the first time or of a survivor having a recurrence, I would find myself overcome with an indescribable darkness.

That's what I felt when Josh called me to tell me about Amy's recurrence. I was devastated. Josh and I were mentally preparing to celebrate my two-year anniversary, but it was hard for me to feel excited about it. Cancer can steal so many of our joys. I'm glad I was able to spend some time with Amy after she received the bad news. I went to see her at a cancer function where she was speaking. I was in absolute awe of her positive outlook and attitude, even in the face of her grim diagnosis. I was once again baffled at how this was happening to her, especially since her initial cancer diagnosis was not nearly as serious as mine had been. But here she was, having to walk through this nightmare all over again.

Amy fought an amazing fight, but it breaks my heart to say she passed away, leaving four precious children behind. She was a gift, an incredible friend and inspiration to me during the hardest time of my life. I hated watching my friends die, and I hated worrying that cancer would ultimately kill me too. I prayed I would live and declare the works of the Lord for a long, long time. I prayed this would not be my ending and that my family would not watch me die the way I'd watched others die. I prayed to live out the calling of Psalm 128, which had been spoken over me so many times, that I would be a fruitful vine in my family.

So Josh and I faced the future together as we walked into my two-year appointment. We knew that would mean more tests, more scans, and more appointments. We also knew it meant talking about potentially starting a family—a battle we knew still awaited us, and one we weren't sure how to win.

CHAPTER 6

ATTEMPTING PREGNANCY AND FIGHTING INFERTILITY

—JOSH—

The time had come.

We were at the tail end of two horrendous years of cancer treatments, surgeries, anxiety, depression, sleeplessness, and grieving. To say we were exhausted at that point would be an understatement. However, despite the pain and struggle of the previous two years, we were about to experience one of the most exciting times of our lives. It was October 2013, the two-year mark of Aly's initial diagnosis. This meant heading back to Houston for a thorough exam. Because Aly's oncologist knew we were thinking about trying to have children, she ordered a full-body scan for this visit. She wanted to be absolutely certain that there was no cancer hiding out in Aly's body as we attempted to get pregnant.

We believed that Aly was completely healed, but there was still a lot of stress around that visit. I was feeling it myself, and I could read it all over Aly's face. She isn't a worrier by nature, but this was a huge appointment for us. Not only did it mean finding out for sure that she was still cancer-free at the two-year mark—a major milestone—but it was the first hurdle we had to overcome to start a family. There was a lot riding on this visit.

It was good to see the team at MD Anderson again. After all, these people helped save my wife's life! I will always owe them a huge debt of gratitude. After a lot of small talk with doctors and nurses, Aly went in for her scan. The next morning we went for our appointment to get the results. The nurse came in and gave an initial report: the doctor had taken a look at the scan and didn't see anything apparent. Aly and I were overwhelmed!

About twenty minutes later, the doctor herself talked to us and confirmed that the scan didn't show anything we should worry about. Being a cautious professional, she said she'd need to wait until the official radiologist report before she signed off on everything, but that report came a short time later and confirmed everything we'd been praying for: Aly was cancer-free at the two-year mark! With that, her chances of recurrence dropped dramatically. It was a huge celebration!

We spent the rest of that appointment talking with the doctor about starting a family and celebrating together. When we were done, the doctor said goodbye, wished us luck, and said she didn't need to see Aly again for six months. *Six months!* After all the constant tests and exams we'd been through, a six-month sabbatical seemed like a dream. From that point on, the doctor only needed to see Aly every six months until she hit her five-year cancer-free milestone. With that, we felt a kind of release from the world of cancer treatment and cancer-related anxiety. Now we were focused on something else: starting a family.

NOT AS FUN AS YOU'D THINK

Years earlier, a buddy complained to me about how "exhausting" it was trying to get pregnant. He and his wife had been trying for a while with no luck. I remember thinking, *Are you kidding me? What are you talking about?* I thought "trying to get pregnant" was another way of saying "having sex all the time." What man in his right mind would complain about that? *Not me,* I smugly thought as my friend whined.

Man, was I wrong. Coming off our two-year appointment at MD Anderson, Aly and I were convinced she'd get pregnant right away. Even though the past two years had been horrible and had taken a huge toll on her body and on both of us emotionally, and despite doctors telling us that the chance of pregnancy was unlikely, we really thought a quick pregnancy would be our next miracle. We imagined introducing everyone to our little miracle baby! That . . . didn't happen. Several months and buckets of tears later, I had a healthy respect for my friend's *exhaustion.* We were shaken by the emotions, timing, pressure, fears, questions, and disappointment that came with each month's negative pregnancy test. The pressure built every month as we started it with hope and ended it with frustration, stuck in a terrible cycle with no end in sight.

Eventually Aly's OB-GYN suggested using an ovulation kit, which would tell her the dates (and even time of day) she was most likely to conceive. She warned us, like the other doctors, about the unlikelihood of us conceiving, but, to us, this was worth a shot. Now it wasn't just sex; it was sex on a rigid schedule. Needless to say, this led to some interesting midday breaks in my workday. It also gave us some hilarious lifelong memories.

In particular I'll never forget the time I had a broken nose when duty called. One afternoon I was playing basketball with my buddies and slammed my face into an opponent's shoulder, hitting the ground with blood gushing out of my nose. I was so dazed I didn't even know where I was for a few minutes. The next day a doctor confirmed that it wasn't just broken; it was broken in *several* places. I had surgery the following day to put the pieces back together, and I went home in more pain (and with more pain meds) than I'd ever had in my life. Aly was a huge support during the whole ordeal—but she also kept me aware of where we were on the ovulation calendar. Sure enough, two days after surgery, still in pain and half-stoned on pain medicine, I came face-to-face with the smiley face on the ovulation kit. It was go time.

—ALY—

Okay, I feel like I should break in at this point. I wasn't *quite* as demanding as Josh remembers. He was half out of his mind on pain pills, remember? Josh was definitely my top priority, but I was consumed with getting pregnant. If you've ever tried to follow an ovulation kit to get pregnant, you know how devastating it can be to discover your partner is out of town or otherwise unavailable when you're ovulating. It means another month you can't get pregnant. But Josh was so kind when I *gently* told him I was ovulating right after his surgery. Despite the pain he was obviously in—not to mention the swollen black eyes and bandages all over his face—he did his best to be there for me. Without going into details, I'll just say that we *tried* . . . but it wasn't happening. I sent him back out to his big comfy chair, where he could fall asleep watching TV, and I lay on the bedroom floor crying. I didn't know if I'd *ever* be able to have a baby, but I had also convinced myself that this would have been *the* month it would have happened if only Josh hadn't gotten hurt. In a weird way, I felt like Josh's accident cost us our only shot at pregnancy. Isn't it nuts how we convince ourselves of these things?

NOT MADE TO BE A MOTHER

After a few more failed months of trying, I had some tests done and discovered that my body wasn't *really* ovulating. It was trying, but it just wasn't happening. Even though we'd been told numerous times that medically it was so unlikely that I would get pregnant, we asked all our doctors to remain hopeful with us. We knew we weren't relying on science to provide for us, but on God and His timing. Thankfully, my doctor stayed positive and was willing to keep working with us. She referred me to a fertility specialist, so we made the appointment and started another waiting game. I was used to all the stress and weird thoughts that popped into my head as I waited for an upcoming doctor's appointment. By this point I was a pro! So as we looked toward the fertility appointment, I found myself wondering if I was even *meant* to be a mother. Maybe God was protecting me from being a mom because He knew I'd be a terrible one. Maybe He knew I wasn't mom material? The one fear I tried not to think about was, *Maybe God isn't letting me get pregnant because He knows I won't live long enough to raise a child.* Whatever the reason, the phrase *maybe I wasn't meant to be a mother* often filled my mind.

In the midst of this whirlwind of fear and doubt, I had a revelation: *I actually wasn't made to be a mother.* It just came to me. It wasn't based in fear or a negative thing at all; it was just a fact. I remembered an email I had received a few months earlier from a friend whose daughter was having fertility issues. She learned she was unable to conceive and was looking into other ways of becoming a mom. My friend shared that her daughter, in a brilliant moment of faith and clarity, said, "God did not necessarily put me on this earth to have babies. I was put here to love and glorify Him in all circumstances." That simple statement hit me like a ton of bricks. I was immediately undone by the power of that truth. I realized that, while I truly believed being a mother is one of the greatest callings on my life, motherhood doesn't define me. *Christ* does.

I had spent so much of my life defined by other things. I was Cyd's daughter, Jessica's sister, and Josh's wife. I was the cancer patient. I was the cancer survivor. I was the PhD student and the therapist. But I came to realize those things did not define me, and neither would being a mom. Instead, I chose to make a list of things that *did* define me. I wanted to be clear on *who* I was and *whose* I was. Here's what I came up with:

I am Aly. *Just Aly.* And *Just Aly* is something incredibly unique. There is no other person like me! I am determined, strong, a child of God, beautiful in His eyes, blameless, goal-oriented, self-motivated, and loving. I'm a wife, a faithful friend, a daughter, a sister, and a niece. I am a hard-working peacemaker, fun-loving, encouraging, and positive. And that's not all!

It's uncomfortable to try to see yourself through God's eyes and make a list of all the wonderful things you are, but it is so important. Try it if you don't believe me! I know that, in that moment and in the midst of our fertility struggle, this was a critical wake-up call in my spirit. God didn't make me to be a mother. He made me to be His precious child and to glorify Him with my life. That's the attitude adjustment I needed before Josh and I took the next steps in our fertility journey, and I'm so grateful God gave me that insight at the perfect time.

ASSESSING FERTILITY OPTIONS

So many emotions flooded my mind as we sat in the fertility doctor's waiting room. I was affirmed in my faith that God made me to be more than a mom, but I still desperately wanted a baby. I sat there praying for direction. I prayed for favor. I prayed for a healthy pregnancy and that we would receive positive news and results.

Once again, we were blessed with a fantastic doctor to walk us through this part of our journey. He was thorough too. He listened patiently as we ran through our cancer story, and he was particularly interested in the type of chemo medicines my oncologist had ordered. He wasn't thrilled to see what they had used. Just by looking at my history, he was pretty sure the chemo drugs had severely damaged my eggs. My oncologist had explained that likelihood at the time we started chemotherapy, so we weren't shocked; but it was still tough to hear the news and see the negative test results now that we were actively trying to have a baby. It was a problem we had deferred as we focused on our cancer fight, and now it was time to face the music.

—JOSH—

The doctor ordered a full round of new bloodwork and gave Aly a new fertility medicine to take while we waited on the test results. After another unsuccessful month of trying, we had our follow-up appointment. When he walked in reading her test results, I could tell he was disappointed but not surprised. He gave us a bunch of numbers we didn't fully understand before dropping the hammer. He told us his assumption had been confirmed: Aly was producing little to no eggs, and there was a good chance that any eggs she *did* have were severely damaged by her cancer treatments. To drive the point home, he said that Aly had begun the menopause process and that it was as though she were trying to get pregnant in her late forties.

I looked at Aly as he gave us the news, and I saw the same devastated face I'd seen during so many other doctor visits. She was crushed. The doctor launched into a speech full of statistics about cancer and infertility, but we cut him off. We didn't want to hear all that. Instead, we simply asked him what he would suggest for us. He explained that everything he told us so far was based only on Aly's bloodwork. The only way to be absolutely sure of his diagnosis would be to actually examine Aly's eggs through a procedure called egg retrieval. If we wanted to do that, though, he said we might as well try in vitro fertilization (IVF), as that would be our best bet at getting pregnant.

This was a lot of information to process from a single office visit. The final punch was him suggesting we begin the process *immediately.* He explained that every month we waited, Aly would lose more and more potentially healthy eggs. Her biological clock was ticking. His next IVF group we could participate in was one month away, so the doctor sent us home to think about it. The two-hour drive home was deathly quiet—but nothing new. I've lost count of how many uncomfortable car rides we've had after doctor appointments, driving down the interstate in silence with life-altering questions looming over us.

—ALY—

That drive home was brutal. Even though I was already feeling comfortable about moving forward with IVF, I was angry that it was this hard. I was confused about why my womb had been so affected. Doctors had warned us about this, but Josh and I believed—*truly believed with everything in us*—that my womb had been protected. We believed my body would grow a baby. We had so many people praying for pregnancy, but it was looking doubtful. However, I was holding out hope that perhaps *this* would be how God would bless me with a baby. We went home, discussed it with our family, prayed a bunch, and then felt peaceful about signing up for the IVF the following month. We figured we should at least reserve our spot, and we could cancel if we changed our minds before then.

While we felt a peace about the procedure, we weren't sure how we'd pay for it. I was shocked by how expensive everything was. Josh and I prayed hard about it, and neither of us were comfortable asking anyone for help. Our friends and family had been so generous during my cancer battle; we didn't want to put this burden on them too. We were able to pay for a portion of IVF through selling one of the rental houses we owned, hosting a big yard sale, and being frugal with our other expenses. However, we were still short. Then, out of the blue, my mom approached us about some money she had saved for us from my dad's life insurance policy. She wanted these funds to be used to fund our remaining fees for IVF. What a huge answered prayer! We were continually amazed at how God provided at every step.

—JOSH—

We had an enormous group of people praying for us as we got ready for this next challenge. Inspired by the incredible faith of a sick man's friends in Mark 2:4–5, Aly had organized a prayer circle she called her "Mark 2 people." These were friends, family members, and people who followed our blog and who committed to pray for us on this journey and specifically in our fertility efforts. We really needed those prayers, because starting the IVF process was overwhelming.

The first week I gave Aly what seemed like ten shots a day. It gave me flashbacks of the shots I had to give her during her cancer treatment. Honestly, all this effort made me angry that she was having to jump through these medical hoops again. We made it through that first week, though, and drove the two hours back to the doctor's office for our first "egg checkup." We were excited; it was the first time we'd be able to see Aly's eggs with an ultrasound, and we'd know for sure what we were dealing with and how well the fertility drugs were working.

As the doctor performed the ultrasound, though, he was visibly disappointed. He spoke to us kindly, but also left little room for doubt about what he was seeing. He explained that the ultrasound showed what he had initially expected, that Aly's eggs were seriously damaged. In fact, he only saw a couple, and they weren't growing like he'd hoped. Since we were only one week into the IVF journey, the doctor suggested we cancel the treatment and look into other options for starting a family. Bottom line: he didn't want us to waste our money on IVF treatments he was pretty sure wouldn't work.

Another two-hour drive home in silence. I knew Aly was hurting as she stared out the window. I was too. Could *anything* in our life be easy? Why was everything so hard? I was frustrated beyond words, but I thought long and hard about what I wanted to say before I opened my mouth. Finally, after praying about it most of the way home, I told Aly what I was thinking. "I think we should continue with the IVF," I said. "I know it's a long shot and the doctor advised against it, but God has done so much more than this in our lives. Let's trust Him for an opportunity to show up in a big way." I could tell she was considering it. I closed with, "Besides, if we stop IVF now, we will always wonder, *What if . . .* What if we *would* have gotten pregnant if we had stuck with it?" We discussed the financial commitment, and I knew it would cost thousands of dollars from the sale of our rent house and Aly's dad's life insurance policy. But I just wasn't ready to give up on IVF yet.

GIVE FROM YOUR PLACE OF PAIN

—ALY—

After hearing Josh out, we decided to stay the course with IVF, though we were both so frustrated and sad. We desperately wanted to give our friends and family an optimistic report, but that never seemed to happen. On top of that, many of our friends started getting pregnant. We were thrilled for them, of course, but it was hard not to hurt for our own loss. I had to learn how to have joy for other people when our situation was anything *but* joyful. I once heard someone say the best thing you can do is to "give from your place of pain." That often feels impossible because our pain makes us feel as though we have nothing left to give. But giving from our pain forces us to take our minds off ourselves, focus on others, and allow ourselves to feel joy for them—no matter what's going on in our own lives.

When you struggle with infertility, it can seem like everyone around you is getting pregnant at the drop of a hat. Many of our friends started having kids while I fought cancer. We rejoiced with them and prayed that we'd join them in parenthood one day. Later, as we struggled through IVF and other friends got pregnant, it was more of a challenge for us. I cried every time I found out someone else was pregnant. I'd like to say they were tears of joy for my friends, but many times they weren't. They were tears of sadness for the loss Josh and I felt. I wallowed in this for a while before I remembered my "not made to be a mother" moment from months earlier.

I realized I had a choice. Would I continue to feel sorry for myself and our current situation, or would I choose to be happy for others and believe God had a plan to grow our family? I chose the second option. It was much easier said than done, of course, but God gave me the strength to show others how happy I was for them. I wanted my friends to feel comfortable talking to me about their pregnancies and how they were feeling, so I had to separate their joy from my heartache. It was hard, though.

THE HIGHS AND LOWS OF IVF

We kept going with IVF, and the day finally came to attempt an egg retrieval. Despite the doctor's doubts, they were able to retrieve not one but *two* eggs—and both were confirmed to be fertilized with Josh's sperm! Success! Finally! We praised God because we knew, no matter what happened, we currently had two Taylor babies. There were still plenty of uphill battles ahead of us, but we let ourselves celebrate this good news.

Five days after getting the good report, we went back to the doctor to have the embryos put back into my body. The doctor called while we were on the road to tell us that one of the embryos had not survived. Josh took the call and was very clear with their office to make sure the embryo really did not survive, not that it just didn't *appear* unhealthy. We would never discard any embryo. But, sadly, it was already lost. We were heartbroken because we had hoped to save one of the embryos for a second Taylor baby later. Now we were down to one. One embryo. One baby. One shot.

I went into the implantation with complete confidence. I knew I was going to be pregnant when this was all over. Like the sick man in Mark 2, I felt the prayers and faith of my friends and family carrying me straight into the healing presence of Jesus. I couldn't wait to proclaim from the rooftops the power of God in working miracles for His children. First, He healed my cancer, and now He was going to give us a miracle baby. It was *going* to happen. I just knew it!

—JOSH—

It would be another week before we found out for sure if Aly was pregnant, but we already knew. Aly had been writing letters to our future baby in a special journal, and we both wrote a note to this baby in Aly's belly. We spoke of the miracle he or she was and how we were believing against all odds. We were truly excited and didn't even entertain the possibility that we *weren't* pregnant. Aly went in for a blood test to confirm the results, and we knew we would get a call from the nurse that afternoon telling us the good news. We built such great relationships with the nurses at the clinic, and they were praying and personally invested in this journey. We all couldn't wait to celebrate this miracle IVF baby together.

As we waited for the phone call, Aly asked me to set up the video camera. We were convinced we were about to get the greatest call of our lives, and we wanted to document the moment to show our child later.

Finally, Aly's phone rang. The fertility clinic's phone number flashed on her screen, and she rushed to tell me to turn on the video camera. Sitting on the couch together, Aly and I answered the call that would change everything. The camera across the room was taking it all in.

"Hello?" Aly answered with a smile in her voice.

When we were greeted by a man's voice, we knew it was the doctor calling us instead of his nurse. I thought, *He wants to give us the good news himself because he can't believe it worked!* There was absolutely no doubt in my mind—until he said one of the most heartbreaking sentences I've ever heard.

"I am so sorry, Aly, but the test is negative. You are not pregnant."

—ALY—

To this day, one of the hardest things to look back on from our whole journey is the video we recorded that day. We forgot all about the camera once the doctor delivered the devastating news that we weren't pregnant.

Watching that little window into one of our darkest moments, you can see me collapse in a heap of tears on Josh's lap. I was so confused. I believed, *really believed*, that my womb had been protected and would produce a miracle baby. We had our Mark 2 friends praying for us. We had promised to give God the glory and shout His praises from the mountaintops. We had been told this was the *only* way we'd be able to have a child, and now that chance was gone. It was over. Our dream of becoming parents was *over*. And we got it all on video.

The news didn't get better in our follow-up appointment a week later. We were looking for options, for some glimmer of hope that there was still something else we could try. The doctor explained that the whole ordeal had proved what he'd initially feared. I had very few eggs left, and they were all severely damaged. Even if I miraculously became pregnant, it would most likely end in a miscarriage. That felt like the end of the line for us, the last stop on the fertility train. However, he had one more suggestion. He said that, despite everything else, I would be an excellent candidate to carry a baby using an egg donor. He explained that I would still be able to carry a baby in my womb and deliver the child myself; the baby just wouldn't have my DNA. We hadn't considered this before, and it was a lot to take in. We went home with a new *huge* question to pray about.

CHAPTER 7

ADOPTION:
THE BEST CHOICE

—ALY—

The egg donation option weighed heavily on us for several days. We prayed about it constantly, trying to discern what God wanted us to do next. During this time Josh started asking a hard (but reasonable) question: "Are we trying too hard for this?" We were stuck trying to figure out what the future held and why we didn't seem able to start a family. We wondered if a family wasn't in the cards for us at all and if it was time to give up this family dream altogether. It was a challenging, terrible time of soul searching for both of us.

In the middle of all this, I heard God speak to me, sending His word directly into my heart. Clear as a bell, I heard Him say, "You aren't *starting* a family. You *already are* one." This was a pivotal moment for me in realizing I already had a wonderful family. The past couple of years had shown me with crystal clarity how blessed I was to have such amazing people in my life—not to mention the absolute best husband in the world. Somewhere along the way we had turned the word *children* into the word *family*, but

God reminded me they aren't the same. He showed me that I didn't necessarily *need* a child to have a family.

Our branch of the Taylor family started on July 22, 2006, when Josh and I said, "I do," but I don't think we understood what that meant at the time. About a year before our IVF failure, we attended a silent auction fund-raiser and accidentally won a family photo session. I say "accidentally" because Josh had just wanted to get the bidding started; he never intended to place the winning bid! We laughed when we won, and we decided to save the photo shoot for later. After all, family photo shoots are for *families*, right? That means kids, two dogs, and a cat. We didn't have any of those, so we set it aside. Why waste a professional family photo session on just the two of us?

A year later, we still hadn't used the session. We hoped to be parents by then or, at least, be pregnant. The unused photo shoot became a symbol of our failed fertility efforts, a reminder that we *weren't* a family. But we were. Josh and I were a wonderful, happy, committed, goofy, blessed family—just the two of us. We'd lost sight of that, of the fact that "just the two of us" is enough.

So, armed with our new understanding of *family*, Josh and I finally scheduled that photo session. It wasn't a maternity shoot, an anniversary shoot, or a massive group shoot with kids, grandkids, and pets running around. It was a session just for the Taylor family circa 2014: Josh and me. And for the first time in a long time, we knew that was enough. If God chose to bless us with kids, that'd be awesome. We were excited for that. But if He didn't for whatever reason, we wanted to be fine with that too.

We didn't come to this place overnight; it was a difficult process to work through. However, God taught us in that season to embrace where we were. That's a message I share loud and clear now: embrace your family *today*. Whoever it is, whatever it looks like, understand that you *have* a family. Don't wait to take your family pictures until life looks the way you *think* it should. Do it now!

—JOSH—

From that point on, we changed our perspective and the language we used about where we were. We weren't *starting* a family; we were *growing* our family. We already were a family, but we wanted it to get bigger!

This was a wonderful season of healing for us. We had been through so much with cancer, surgeries, infertility, and failed IVF. Neither of us were ready to rush into anything, so we took a break. In that time of rest, God entered in and reset our hearts in a meaningful way. By the time the fertility clinic called us with a potential egg donor match, Aly and I had a shared peace about saying no. On the one hand, it was a big leap of faith to turn down an opportunity to have a child; on the other, we were sure this wasn't what God wanted for us and we didn't want our desire for a child to lead us out of step with His will. We thanked the fertility clinic for their help and commitment to us, but we turned them down and continued praying about which direction to go next.

IT WAS ADOPTION ALL ALONG

All through our journey, people asked us if we'd ever consider adoption. The answer was an immediate yes; we both always wanted to adopt a child. However, we also believed strongly that God had protected Aly's womb. That was clear in our minds, so we were confused about why we were having so much trouble getting pregnant. Even after the failed IVF, we still believed God could work a miracle in Aly's body, allowing her to have a child naturally. While we never considered adoption as second best, we also didn't want to allow adoption to cut short our belief in God's ability to produce a child through Aly.

We both spent a lot of time praying about adoption during this time, but we were scared to bring it up with each other. I knew adoption was becoming a greater focus for me, but I didn't want to influence Aly. I found out later that she felt the same way! We didn't realize that God was leading both of us toward adoption. And as we discovered shortly thereafter, His timing, as always, was perfect.

—ALY—

As we were praying for direction in how to grow our family, my cousin reached out to me out of the blue and asked if Josh and I wanted to adopt. I told her we were praying about the timing, but that we both wanted to at some point. That gave her the green light to start a conversation that changed our lives forever. My cousin, an OB-GYN nurse, explained that a pregnant teenage girl had recently come into their office. As she got to know the girl, something about her and her boyfriend reminded her of me and Josh. When the expectant mother admitted that she wasn't sure if she'd be able to keep the child and mentioned adoption as a possibility, my cousin thought of us.

As I listened to this news, something in my spirit was immediately drawn to this couple and this baby. Everything in me wanted to reply, "Yes! Yes, we'll take that baby!" However, I had no idea where Josh was emotionally and how he was feeling about everything. As Josh said, we weren't actively talking about adoption much because we didn't want to put any more pressure on each other. Plus, we were still healing from the news that I'd likely never have a biological child. Things were calming down a bit for us, and I didn't want to drop this new bomb on him. However, I also didn't want to miss out on what might be a huge God moment, so I decided to go to his office that day and *casually* mention the call from my cousin. Sure, that seems silly; how do you casually mention that someone wants to know if you'll adopt a baby? I was just trying to feel him out to see how he'd respond.

Let's just say there was *nothing* casual about this conversation with Josh. I have never seen him more certain about anything in his life! I could barely get the whole story out of my mouth before he exclaimed, "Yes, of course we're interested!" I just about peed my pants! This was the moment I realized Josh was just as ready as I was to move forward with the idea of adopting. I had all these thoughts and fears of us not being on the same page, but he was the one willing to just jump in. I was the one who was overthinking everything!

With Josh's agreement and after lots of prayer, I was all in. The first step was to create a profile book, a collection of pictures and information about ourselves that the prospective birth family could use to get to know us. I put that book together in a single night! I wanted to get it to my cousin as soon as possible so she'd have it the next time she saw the pregnant teen. I was so excited to think about this young girl and wondered if she was carrying *our* baby. Now all we could do was wait.

A month later we found out that the girl decided to keep her baby, which we learned was a little boy. Thankfully, we were never officially matched with this couple, but I'd be lying if I said I hadn't started picturing us adopting this baby. Learning this wasn't *our* child was a disappointment, but the whole experience gave us an incredible gift: it showed us how excited we were to start the adoption process. Isn't it funny how God puts different situations in your life to prepare you for *the* situation? It really is true that every no prepares you for a bigger yes.

Josh and I were convinced now that adoption was how God wanted to grow our family, but we were clueless about how to start. So I went into deep research mode, reading everything I could find and talking to everyone we knew who had adopted. I discovered there are several ways to adopt with different agencies, states, processes, and even different countries. How would I know which route was best for us? Once again I found myself confused and wishing God would write the answer on the wall for us. This was a tense time of research and discovery, but I didn't feel weighed down by the pressure at all. In fact, I felt downright giddy. It dawned on me that I was pregnant in a way. I was *adoption pregnant*. I didn't know if I'd be pregnant for a day, three months, or three years, but I was pregnant. It's the only way I can describe how I felt at the time.

—JOSH—

The more we talked about and researched adoption, the more excited we got. Honestly, we felt silly for doing IVF and for trying so hard to get pregnant. Not that there's anything wrong with IVF; I know it's the right choice for many families. For us, though, it became clear that adoption had been the answer all along. That said, I was still scared. I think if Aly had gotten pregnant, I would have been scared but would have fully embraced it—even though there would have been a huge chance of having a miscarriage. As scary as a pregnancy would have been, though, I think adoption scared me more. I could feel myself wanting to fully dive into the process, but I also felt like I needed to protect myself a little.

Aly, on the other hand, was going full steam ahead and talking to anyone and everyone she could think of who could help her understand how adoption works. Every night she'd mention an agency she found or someone she talked to. This made me a bit nervous. I didn't want to rain on her parade, but at the same time I didn't want her to get hurt again. I didn't know how much more bad news we could take.

God went to work on my fear. One night while I was on a hunting trip, I felt the Lord tell me I needed to let Aly enjoy and fully embrace this process. My protective nature had not allowed me to go all in yet, and I realized I was preventing Aly from experiencing what most women go through when they're pregnant. Yes, it was scary; but if we were going to do this, we needed to do it all the way—together. When I got home I apologized to Aly for being so overprotective, and I promised to do everything I could to help her experience every part of her adoption pregnancy.

GOD FUNDS WHAT HE FAVORS

With both of us on the same page and fully committed to the adoption process, it was time to consider some practical matters. The past few years had been really, *really* expensive. The medical bills from Aly's treatments had been significant, and we had just spent thousands more on IVF treatments. If adoption was God's plan for us, we knew He'd have to provide a way to make it happen. Soon after, as we were researching fund-raising options, a friend told Aly something that changed how we viewed the financial side of adoption. She said, "God funds what He favors." That simple statement took a lot of the pressure off us. We knew God had called us to adopt, and we knew He favored adoption. After all, Ephesians 1:5 says that *He* has adopted *us*! "He predestined us for adoption to sonship through Jesus Christ, in accordance with his pleasure and will." God had shown us time and again that He's bigger than our financial obstacles, and we trusted Him to do it again. But how would He fund it?

—ALY—

During this time Josh and I were talking about wanting to share our story more. We still updated the blog every now and then, but we felt a growing responsibility to tell people more about what God had done in our lives. That's when lightning struck: What if we started doing some public speaking and shared our testimony? We could put any money we made from that toward our adoption. That way we could be an encouragement to others and try to get a little extra money for our adoption without having to ask for donations. Genius!

Over the next few months, we were blessed with several opportunities to speak at breast cancer events, churches, hospitals, universities, and many other different events around the country. We also renewed our commitment to writing. The blog had been a big source of encouragement for us during my cancer fight; not only was it therapeutic for us in writing it, but we knew it had been a blessing for other cancer patients who followed along with our journey.

I remembered how disappointed I was the day I looked through the cancer section of the local bookstore, and I began to dream about writing a book for women facing their own cancer diagnosis. I thought, *Can I write a book? And if I did, would anyone read it?* We looked into different publishing options and decided to go for it. Since any sales of the book would go toward our adoption fund, we went the self-publishing route. That made things go a lot faster with fewer complications. I started writing, and soon after we released my first book, *How Cancer Made Me a Mommy.* The sales of that little book, along with our speaking engagements, funded one-third of our adoption!

Don't be discouraged by finances if you are considering adopting or are in the adoption process. There are fund-raising options all around you. It may be a typical fund-raiser like selling a T-shirt or having a garage sale, but it could be something you haven't considered yet. Maybe it's telling your story of how you came to the decision to adopt. It may be writing a book. If you are crafty, it might be selling crafts. If you cut grass, it could be mowing yards. Just look at your life and see what you can do—using your gifts and talents—to help raise money to bring your baby home.

MAKING IT OFFICIAL

As we got serious about raising money and our excitement about adoption grew, we finally landed on an adoption attorney. She lived in our area, and we knew several people who had had great experiences with her. We agreed we'd start the formal process at the start of 2015. We had our research, we had a plan, we had a start date, and we had a lawyer. Finally, we were making progress! As 2014 came to a close, Josh and I were ready to jump into action at the start of the new year.

—JOSH—

With all our ducks in a row, Aly and I began winding down for the year and were looking forward to a little break. We definitely needed to catch our breath. That didn't stop Aly from flexing her research muscles, of course, and she kept talking to different adoption families to hear their stories. One of the people she spoke to was my childhood babysitter, Deneé, who had recently adopted through a lawyer we hadn't learned of in our research yet. Our friend told Aly all about her attorney and the process he used, and it seemed interesting. Instead of making a profile that is sent to all birth mothers to review and decide if we were a right fit, this attorney kept an email list of potential adoptive parents and sent out an email that contained information about birth mothers looking for someone to adopt the babies they were carrying. Potential adoptive parents could then apply to a specific case for a birth mother to review. This method seemed to help streamline a very emotional and intense process. Even though we'd decided on another attorney, we didn't see any harm in signing up for his email list. So we passed along our information and didn't think much else of it.

Soon afterward, I came home from work and saw Aly sitting on the couch with the biggest smile on her face. She said, "Josh, you *have* to read this email." It was the first email she'd received from our friend's adoption attorney. As we read the message together, I could tell she felt like this case was a perfect match for us. We'd already been down this road when her cousin reached out about the pregnant teen a few months earlier, but this felt different. As I read through the profile of this birth mother, it was clear she was amazing. However, the part that really stood out to us was what the birth mother wrote about the type of family she was hoping to find to raise the baby she was carrying. It was as though she was describing Aly and me. We both got chills and wondered what we should do next.

We contacted the attorney's office and learned that we now needed to submit an application for the birth mother to review. She would go through all the applications and hopefully choose the adoptive family. Aly and I liked how this attorney worked. His system seemed geared to leading birth families and adoptive families into the best decisions by working together. He also suggested that once a family was chosen the prospective parents should meet with the birth family in person to make sure everyone felt good about the decision. That part scared me, but I could see the wisdom in it.

The application deadline for this particular case was that week, so we knew we had to hurry if we were interested.

—ALY—

This case caught us off guard. We thought we had everything figured out, but then, out of the blue, here was what seemed like a perfect opportunity. Even though we were planning to sign up with the other attorney a few weeks later, we decided to apply for this one case. I said, "If we aren't chosen, we'll just move forward with our plan." So that's what we did. We turned in an application for this child—along with twenty-two other couples—and were told we'd have an answer in a week.

We tried to go about everyday life, but of course we were anxious to hear if we had been chosen. Thankfully, it was Christmastime, and we were busy with family parties, work get-togethers, and all things Christmas. One afternoon, as I was on my way home after some gift shopping, I got a phone call from an out-of-state number I'd never seen before. It quickly dawned on me that it must be the attorney. We had never spoken to him, so it was a bit surreal. I answered, and he said, "Is this Mrs. Taylor?" I said yes, and he continued, "My name is [attorney], and I have your husband on the other line." My heart was about to beat out of my chest. I was hanging on every word—but then the call dropped! Total freak-out. I couldn't believe what was happening, but all I could do was sit there and wait for the phone to ring again.

Finally, the attorney called back and I could hear Josh on the line as well. That's when we heard the most beautiful news of our lives: "Mr. and Mrs. Taylor, congratulations! The birth mother chose you!" I was stunned. I couldn't speak. I could tell Josh felt the same way, because neither of us said anything. We managed to get the necessary details before hanging up the phone right as I arrived at our apartment. I ran through the front door and straight into Josh's arms. We were truly, officially *adoption pregnant*!

The attorney had given us the birth mother's name and contact information, and he suggested we all meet as soon as possible to confirm our desire to move forward with the adoption. The baby was a girl, and the birth mother was due in March—just three months away. There was no time to waste! We immediately booked plane tickets and made plans to meet the woman who was carrying—*gulp*—our daughter.

MEETING THE BIRTH FAMILY

—JOSH—

Three days later, we were waiting for the okay to walk into a restaurant states away from our home to meet the birth mother. The adoption counselor wanted to talk to her first, and he said he'd text when she was ready for us. What a weird moment. We'd picked up a small gift for her, but we kept second-guessing our decision to give it to her. We didn't want to overwhelm her, but we also didn't want to seem too casual about everything. There really aren't any rules for what to do or say when you meet the woman who's carrying your baby.

I circled the Panera Bread parking lot a minimum of fifty times waiting on that text. My stomach was in knots, and it started to hit me what was about to happen. We had no clue what the mom even looked like. She would recognize us from our picture on the application, but we hadn't seen a picture of her. *If all else fails*, I thought, *we'll just look for the lady who's six months pregnant!*

The counselor finally texted, and we parked the car, took a breath, and went inside. Fortunately, we didn't have to depend on our foolproof look-for-the-pregnant-lady plan, as the counselor met us at the door and led us to the table. The birth mother, whom we'll call Karen (not her real name) throughout the rest of the book, was sitting with a family member and could not have been warmer or kinder to us. As weird as it was for us, I can't imagine how it must have felt for her to sit there meeting the strangers she was supposed to entrust with the child growing inside her. As we sat down and started talking, everything in me wanted to make her feel more at ease, but my voice wasn't cooperating. My nerves got the best of me, and I probably didn't say ten words the whole time. I'm so glad Aly was there to make a good impression!

—ALY—

This was one of the first times I'd ever seen Josh completely freeze up. All our friends and family know that Josh is the more outgoing of the two of us. Not that day. He sat there almost completely silent while Karen and I talked the entire time. She and I clicked immediately; we both started crying as soon as we sat down. I had the strangest sensation of a special connection with her right from the start. We talked for two hours straight about everything from adoption to sports teams to family to her future plans. It was so strange to meet a new friend, all the while knowing she was carrying the baby we had prayed so hard and long for.

The counselor stayed with us the whole time, asking us questions and guiding us through what the process would look like. He asked about the birth and if Karen wanted us to be in the room when the baby was born. Karen invited us inside the delivery room for the birth, which was a huge blessing. I had been praying for that since we first started considering adoption. It was such a gift to know we would be there for this baby's very first breath. The counselor also asked about what level of contact, if any, we would like to have with Karen after the birth and what she would prefer, and what we each wanted out of the relationship. We didn't have all the answers that day, but we agreed to take things one day at a time and always strive to do the best thing for this precious child.

As we ended the meeting that day, we expressed our love and appreciation to Karen, and we told her she was a direct answer to prayer for us. We stressed how brave she was and acknowledged how hard we knew this decision must have been for her. She told us that she wanted to do what was best for this baby, and she knew she'd be unable to care for the child herself. I was humbled by this young woman's poise and courage. I knew I was witnessing the most incredible act of selfless love imaginable. Karen and I hugged and cried as we left the restaurant. It was as though we had just had dinner with an old friend. This wasn't an old friend, however; this was the woman carrying our baby!

—JOSH—

Watching Aly connect with this young woman was awe-inspiring. Under normal circumstances, these two ladies would have had little in common. They had vastly different backgrounds and experiences, but they shared a special, intimate, immediate bond from the moment Aly and I walked in. Even coming from seemingly different worlds, they were quite similar in that they were both kind, loving, funny, and warm. Speaking as a proud husband, I think this is just one of the many reasons why Aly is such an amazing therapist. She knows how to connect with people, and she genuinely loves them. I was so grateful to her for leading the charge to forge such a wonderful relationship with the birth mother.

And yes, I didn't speak most of the time. I can't explain what happened. At one point Karen even looked me in the eye and joked, "Josh, do you talk?" I laughed and said yes . . . and then kept quiet. I guess the whole experience was just a bit much for me. As we got back in the car that day, the only word I can use to describe how I felt is *thankful*. We were thankful for this brave woman's decision, thankful for God connecting us to her, and thankful that the meeting had gone better than we could have expected. We loved this woman. She was our hero!

We were barely back on the road when the attorney called. Karen had already called him and told him how much she loved us. He wanted to confirm with us that we still wanted to move forward with the adoption, and we couldn't say yes fast enough. What a day!

—ALY—

Driving away from that Panera Bread meeting, we knew we had three months to prepare for this beautiful baby, and we decided to go all in on experiencing this time just as we would if I was pregnant. Sure, something could go wrong, but we believed God wanted us to celebrate. At any point in the process—up to and even after the baby was born—the adoption could fall apart. But an actual pregnancy has risks too. That doesn't stop people from having baby showers, setting up a nursery, getting the house ready, picking baby names, and making other plans and preparations. So we had a gender-reveal party and a baby shower. We got hand-me-downs from friends. We bought a crib and got everything together for her nursery. We picked her name—Genevieve Rose, which means "chosen angel." We knew this child was an angel and that she had been chosen for us just as a rose is picked from a bush. She was our chosen, loved, beautiful, little angel. We couldn't wait to bring her home!

The next few months flew by as we anxiously prepared to meet our baby girl. We thought the hard part was over. We were finally matched and had everything planned. All that was left was to wait for the call that the birth mother was in labor. Oh, if it had only been that simple. Apparently nothing ever comes too easily or simply for us.

CHAPTER 8

OUR GENEVIEVE: OUR FIRST TRUE MIRACLE

—ALY—

The wait for Genevieve was somehow crazy fast and slow as molasses at the same time. I was working as a school counselor and had already arranged maternity leave for when we brought her home, but I was getting anxious. *What if Karen goes into labor early? What if I miss Genevieve's birth? What if there are complications late in the pregnancy?* Josh and I lived twelve hours away from Karen, and I started to worry that we wouldn't be able to get there in time for any last-minute issues—especially since Karen had started showing signs of early labor at just thirty-four weeks.

Josh and I discussed our options, and we decided it'd be best if I could go to be with Karen earlier than we originally planned. I worked it out with my boss, and he agreed to let me start my maternity leave a few weeks early. That meant I'd lose the time on the back end after the baby was born, but it was still worth it to me to ensure I'd be there for the delivery. Besides, I had summers off from work, so I knew I'd have plenty of time to spend with my baby girl.

Karen was due on March 22, but I was able to temporarily move to her state at the end of February. From that point on, I was on baby watch. It's crazy to think of how many connections we had in so many different states, and what a blessing these connections turned out to be. That month I stayed in an acquaintance's condo, a friend's apartment, and the home of a sorority sister's father. We weren't especially close to these people before all this, but they were so gracious in letting us impose on them during this critical time in our lives.

These wonderful people inspired Josh and me to always open our own home to people in need. Once you've been on the receiving end of that kind of grace and generosity, you want to pay it forward whenever and however you can. That experience really gave us a passion for hosting and hospitality, and we'll always be grateful for those acts of kindness.

I had no idea how much of a blessing it would be for me to be there so early. I thought I was just going to lay low and wait for Genevieve to arrive. I had no idea how important it would be for me to be there those few weeks before she was born.

—JOSH—

Sending Aly a little early gave us a huge sense of peace and relief, and I followed a week later. We were so excited that Karen was going to allow us to be in the delivery room that we couldn't imagine *not* being there simply because we lived so far away.

We kept Karen informed of where we were and what we were doing, but we tried not to impose on her and her family during this monumental time in their lives. However, as we talked, we realized that transportation was a big issue for Karen. She didn't always have access to a car or a ride, so we offered to shuttle her around to her doctor appointments. I can't explain how much of a blessing that was for all of us. Aly and I were able to sit in on these final few doctor visits and hear firsthand what was going on with

Genevieve, and we were able to spend unexpected quality time with Karen. We went out to lunch together several times and got to know each other really well. The three of us realized that we would always be connected from that moment on, so we understood the importance of developing that bond.

One day after an appointment, I took Aly and Karen to get pedicures. The nail technicians gave us some funny looks and asked if we were friends or family. We all looked at each other and said, "Family." It was true. Karen had become part of our family, and she was giving us the most precious gift we ever could have received.

—ALY—

That time with Karen is one of the highlights of my life. The bond we forged over those weeks was critical to our relationship and our level of trust with each other. She was no longer a stranger who was about to give birth to my daughter; she was family. I loved her and had so much respect for her selfless decision to do what was best for the baby. She opened up to us too. She told me how hard it was for her to think about handing Genevieve over to us, but she always assured us that she was 100 percent confident it was the right decision. In her mind, Josh and I were this child's parents. So even though I knew there was a big chance she could have second thoughts, the fact that we were having open and honest communication about the adoption gave me a sense of peace and security.

SHE'S COMING!

At Karen's thirty-eight-week mark, the doctor told us it would still be a while and that we should all relax a little bit. Josh and I took his advice and decided to take a break from the nonstop pressure of always being ready to run to the hospital at a moment's notice. We unpacked our hospital bag (because we knew we'd need those clothes over the next few days), did some shopping, and then relaxed for the rest of that afternoon. Later we decided to ride our bikes to the Starbucks down the road. We had such a great time! Until, that is, I wrecked my bike. I was so embarrassed. There I was, a grown woman sitting next to a crashed bike with tears streaming down my face and blood pouring out of my chin. Plus, Josh and I couldn't stop laughing. We were such a sight to see.

We got back to the house and, as I was trying to clean up the big scrape on my chin, Karen's mother called. You guessed it: her water broke! Curse the doctor's orders to relax! Josh flew around the house like a maniac, repacking the hospital bag and putting away all the groceries we had bought earlier. I did my best to stay calm and run through my mental to-do list that I'd been preparing for the past three months. I felt like I was about to burst, but he told me later how weirdly calm I seemed at the time. In fact, he said he was super annoyed as I went about my careful tasks when all he wanted to do was jump in the car and race to the hospital like Jeff Gordon. Anyway, with my few jobs done, I took a quick shower, tried covering my scraped chin with some cover-up, and told Josh I was ready. It was time to go meet our daughter.

—JOSH—

As soon as we got to the hospital and found out Karen's room number, the nurses showed us right back. Karen had already given us permission to be there with her, and the hospital staff had been told about our relationship. Karen was relieved to see us, and we were thrilled to be there on time. She had just been given her epidural, so she was feeling pretty good. We waited together and talked a bit as things progressed. It was surreal to sit in the delivery room of a woman who wasn't my wife knowing she was about to give birth to my daughter!

About 10:00 p.m., Aly stepped out to run to the bathroom. Literally the moment she walked out, the doctor checked Karen and said, "She's completely dialated. It's time to go." After everything we'd done to make sure we were there for the birth, Aly wasn't in the room!

I ran down the hallway after her, yelling, "Baby! Hurry! Come back in here! She's about to push!" We got back in the room just in time. Aly went straight into birthing coach mode. She held Karen's hair back and encouraged her as she pushed. I was a little dazed at first, to be honest. After thinking about it for several months, I still wasn't sure how I would feel watching a woman—not my wife—push out my baby. I think I would have been freaked out enough as a new dad watching my own wife do this, but now I was supposed to stand there and watch someone I'd only known a few months do it?

Here's the kicker, though. Standing in that delivery room, I knew it was *my baby* in there. This wasn't a stranger's birth; this was *my daughter's* birth. I honestly don't think I would have felt any different if it had been Aly lying on that table. I was a little surprised that I wasn't grossed out at all. Instead, I was amazed at what I was witnessing. I was standing there watching my child enter the world. I was watching my wife become a mother. This was something we had always dreamed about, always talked about . . . but it had been hard to hold on to that dream over the years. After so many trials and heartaches and bad hospital visits, I realized I'd let myself start to doubt whether this moment would ever come. But here it was, playing out right in front of me. I was witnessing a miracle, and an uncontrollable wave of emotion crashed into me. I was a mess.

—ALY—

Genevieve was perfect. Absolutely beautiful and perfect. Her temperature was a little low, so they had to put her under a lamp to warm her up. I was eager to hold her, but I was also making sure Karen was feeling okay. Karen's mother and a few other family members were there, and we were all embracing and crying and celebrating Genevieve's arrival.

Finally, the nurses said Genevieve was ready to be held. I wanted to jump up and grab that baby as quickly as possible, but I knew I needed to be considerate of the birth family. I asked, "Can I hold her?" and they all smiled and said yes. So the nurse put my baby girl in my arms for the first time. I got to hold her and feed her; it was the most perfect moment of my entire life.

Josh also took a turn holding her. He tried to feed her but Genevieve wouldn't drink from her bottle well for anyone other than me. I felt this swell of motherhood come over me. Suddenly, everything just came naturally for me, and I felt myself become immediately attached to her. I couldn't imagine being more connected to this little girl if I had been the one to give birth to her. She was our gift. Our promise. Our beautiful chosen rose and angel. Our Genevieve.

THE CRITICAL MOMENT

—JOSH—

The birth experience could not have been better. Karen and her family were incredible to us, and Aly and I never felt out of place the whole time. However, we also tried to be aware of the sensitivities at play. Our attorney had advised us to make sure the birth family had plenty of time with the baby. As much as we wanted to have Genevieve all to ourselves, we knew these were the last moments they'd have with her, and we wanted to be respectful of that. So we agreed to let them have a few hours with her that night and said we'd talk to them in the morning.

The hospital gave Aly and me a room right down the hall from Karen, so we settled in for the night and tried to get some rest. We weren't sure if the baby would be in the nursery that night or in the room with the family, so we set our alarm to go off every hour and took turns going out to see if she was in the nursery. After a long night of interruptions, morning finally came and the birth family called for us to come get her. We were soaking up every minute with her. She was absolutely stunning with a full head of dark hair. Oddly enough, the birth family kept commenting on how much she looked like me! It meant a great deal to us that they were giving us so much time with her and not being possessive of her or threatened by us. We sat in our hospital room, now a family of three—Aly, Genevieve, and me—as Aly and I took in every expression, gurgle, swaddle wrap, diaper change, and bottle feeding.

—ALY—

The morning we spent in the hospital room with her was heaven. Absolute heaven. I'd never been so happy! However, I knew from experience that joy can turn to sorrow at the drop of a hat when you're sitting in a hospital room. I didn't realize it yet, but I was about to get a painful reminder of that.

The birth grandmother called, and I picked up the phone. We had spent so much time together that month that the two of us immediately started chatting about the events of the day and how sweet Genevieve was. As the conversation went along, she mentioned that they were trying to find a car seat they could use. I said, "Oh, you guys don't have to worry about that! We have a car seat. We have everything Genevieve needs!" Something didn't feel right, though. A voice in the back of my head started asking, *Why are they looking for a car seat?* That's the instant everything changed.

She explained that Karen was having second thoughts and was trying to figure out a way she could keep the baby. I thought I'd heard her incorrectly. I sat there in complete silence; I had no words. What was I supposed to say? Genevieve was literally asleep in my arms as we were having this conversation! This was *my* daughter! I'd spent every second telling her that I was her mother and pouring out my entire heart to her, and now we were faced with the possibility that she wouldn't be ours? Somehow God gave me grace and compassion in that moment, and I spoke kindly to the birth grandmother.

I told her that I couldn't imagine what they were feeling and that we would talk when they got back to the hospital. In the meantime, I said, we'd be there caring for Genevieve.

—JOSH—

Aly hung up the phone and told me everything that was said. I thought she was overreacting. I reminded her that we knew Karen would struggle with the decision. I told her to take a breath and trust that everything would be okay. But Aly was completely white. She could barely speak, and I knew she was about to lose it. I remember thinking to myself how emotional everyone was and how certain I was that Aly or the grandmother was exaggerating the seriousness of the situation. After all, we'd all spent months preparing for this. Genevieve was our daughter. Nothing was going to change that. I knew I just had to wait for everyone to calm down. Oh, how wrong I was.

A few minutes later, I got a call from our adoption attorney and the counselor. They confirmed our worst fears: the birth mother had changed her mind and was trying to parent Genevieve. I couldn't believe it. How did we get here? After so much time, planning, preparation, and prayer, none of this made sense. This was my daughter we were talking about. I was her daddy. I couldn't imagine stepping aside and letting someone else drive her home and raise her. But there was nothing we could do except wait and pray—the two things that drove us crazy during so much of Aly's cancer battle. We sat there crying in the hospital room with Genevieve, still pouring our hearts out to her and connecting with her on every level, fully knowing that it was now likely the Taylor family was returning to Louisiana as a family of two.

—ALY—

Numb. Totally, completely numb. My mind couldn't comprehend what was happening. My friends say I dropped off the map at that point. Until that phone call from the birth grandmother, I had been texting updates and pictures of Genevieve nonstop. As soon as I got that call, though, I cut off all contact. I didn't even reach out to update them on what was going on. I couldn't do anything or think about anything except the baby girl who was still in my arms. I was totally focused on my pain and worrying about this child's future. Karen continued to say the best thing for Genevieve would be to go with Josh and me, but she also kept saying she wanted to keep her. It was confusing. The thought of going home without my daughter crippled me.

We kept getting updates from the birth family, but every phone call, text, and message through the grapevine made us more and more convinced that we were going home without our baby. Karen was discharged from the hospital and went home on Saturday, but adoption protocols had Genevieve staying there until Monday. We told the family that we'd be there through Monday, the day Karen would have to sign the papers if she was going through with the adoption. She allowed us to stay at the hospital with Genevieve, which we were grateful for, but she also made it clear she was trying to find a way to keep her. It was such a tense weekend, and everyone was waiting for Monday, which would be the final decision day.

As soon as Karen went into labor, Josh and I had called our parents, who then started the long trek to see their granddaughter. When they arrived we had to greet them with the news that the adoption seemed to be falling apart. They were devastated. They thought they were there to meet their granddaughter! As a family we'd been through so much together. Cancer. Infertility. And now what seemed to be a failed adoption.

All the waiting was eating me alive. Josh and I soaked up every minute we could spend with Genevieve that weekend. We studied her every move, watched her every breath, and laughed at her every sound. There was nothing else we could do, though. This whole nightmare—the outcome of which would change our entire lives—was totally out of our hands. It was the most painful, stressful few days of my life—and that's saying *a lot*. All we could do, though, was spend time with the bundle of joy in our arms and fall deeper and deeper in love with her, and that's what we did.

Josh was amazing during this time. I know he was dying inside, too, but he took such wonderful care of me and Genevieve. He handled all the communication with everyone and did his best to keep me sane. Over and over, he told me, "We just have to stay here and fight and trust God for what's best." He read Scripture to me, praying 2 Corinthians 12:9 over us: "He said to me, 'My grace is sufficient for you, for my power is made perfect in weakness.' Therefore I will boast all the more gladly about my weaknesses, so that Christ's power may rest on me." Goodness, we were weak, and we needed Christ's power. We clung to each other and to our daughter, making the most of our time in that little hospital room.

Monday finally arrived. When Karen got to the hospital, I asked for a moment alone with her, as we hadn't had a chance to talk one-on-one. I asked her how she was feeling, hoping she'd had a revelation over the past few days. Instead, she replied, "Aly, I don't think I can go through with the adoption. I am going to try to keep her." I fought back my sobs, but I was also overcome with compassion for this young woman. I had never given birth before, so I couldn't imagine what she was going through, facing the prospect of handing over this baby to another family forever. I hugged her and wanted to convince her of all the reasons she had previously given us for choosing adoption, but I didn't. I just cried with her and held her.

This was the moment when I lost all hope. Genevieve wasn't going to be ours after all. I couldn't believe it. I had no idea how I would recover from this. I knew God restores, and I knew He could do it, but I had never felt *this* broken. Healing seemed impossible. I knew I would have a hole in my heart that would last a lifetime.

Karen and I walked down what seemed like the longest hallway in the world to tell her mom and Josh that Karen had made her final decision. She wasn't going through with the adoption. Karen's mother was *not* in favor of this decision. She knew adoption was the best choice for everyone—especially the baby—but she was also trying to be compassionate and empathetic toward her daughter. Genevieve was in the nursery and we definitely wanted to tell her goodbye, but Josh asked if we could pray with them one last time before we went our separate ways for good.

—JOSH—

I felt an undeniable urge to pray for Karen and her mother. As devastated as we were for ourselves, we knew we had to pray for Genevieve's birth family. We had dreamed of the day we'd be able to tell our daughter about Jesus Christ, but now we knew that responsibility would fall on Karen and her family. So I wanted to pray over them and bless them before we left. As I prayed, I spoke words of value. Karen had a rough background, and I knew she struggled with a sense of worthiness. I prayed she would know how loved she was. I told her she was a beloved child of the King. I prayed for favor, blessing, wisdom, and the fruit of the Spirit. I prayed for it all. We finished praying, hugged, and expressed our love for each other. I knew this was the last time we'd be together. It was brutal, but the Holy Spirit was there, binding us all together.

—ALY—

I need to be real here. While Josh was feeling the Holy Spirit's presence, I was feeling a whole bunch of nothing. All I wanted to do was crawl into a hole and never come out. The truth is, I don't remember much about Josh's prayer at all. I remember a sense that the Spirit was speaking through him, but I felt trapped behind a wall of emotion. My main focus at the time was getting out of the hospital without completely falling apart.

After Josh ended his prayer and we all started saying goodbye, I saw something I'd never seen before. Peace—a perfect, angelic peace—flooded

Karen's face. She had a glow about her all of a sudden. She looked more beautiful than I had ever seen her, and she is a beautiful woman. It seemed as though she wanted to say something, but she couldn't get the words out. Finally, she spoke and started telling us about a time in her life when she felt the Lord speak to her. She told us how powerful that moment was for her and how she'd always remembered what His presence felt like. Then she said the words I never thought I'd hear her say.

"God just spoke to me again," she said. "He told me that you are Genevieve's parents. There isn't a doubt in my mind. She is your daughter."

What? I thought I might fall on the floor in convulsions from the emotional roller coaster we'd just been on. But Karen wasn't overcome with emotion at all. She was speaking plainly with a rock-solid voice. She told us to go and love on Genevieve in the nursery while she called the attorney to get the papers ready. This was really happening! God had stepped in and given her the peace she needed to fully let go of Genevieve, to entrust her child to us forever. It was in every sense of the word a *miracle*. God had saved our family, just as powerfully and wondrously as He had saved my life.

As Karen and her mother left the waiting room, I completely lost it. I sobbed louder than I ever had before. I didn't care how loud I was, how much of a scene I was making, or how ugly I looked. I was too overjoyed to care.

—JOSH—

We checked in with the attorney and counselor, and they confirmed that the papers were on their way. A short while later, we sat down with Karen, the attorney, and the counselor, and Karen signed everything, making the adoption official. I could not get over the change we saw in her whole presence that day. Even as she signed the adoption paperwork, she was all smiles. She joked with us, and she called us Mom and Dad the rest of the day. With all the surprises and miracles we'd seen throughout Aly's fight with cancer, I had never seen anything like Karen's transformation. There is no doubt that God showed up in that hospital waiting room that day, and I could not be more grateful for the grace and courage He gave Genevieve's birth mother.

—ALY—

Just like that, I was officially a mommy. But the truth is nothing really changed for me emotionally toward Genevieve once papers were signed. I had already given her all of me from the moment we were matched with her. I am so thankful I didn't hold back bonding with her until she was "officially" ours. We had just witnessed a genuine miracle, and now, finally and forever, I was Genevieve's mommy. Our hearts, our home, and our family were full, and we didn't think life could get any more perfect than it was as we drove away from the hospital that day.

Little did we know that God had even more surprising miracles in store for us, which we'd discover soon enough.

CHAPTER 9

OUR FAMILY GROWS AGAIN

—JOSH—

Genevieve Rose Taylor was an absolute dream baby. Watching her sleep in her crib, seeing her little tummy rise and fall with each breath, it was as if Aly's cancer started to make sense for the first time. As hard as it was for us to admit or even acknowledge that cancer had taken Aly's fertility, had it not, we may not have had our Genevieve—and we simply cannot fathom life with her. So, for that, cancer . . . thank you for taking my wife's fertility.

Bringing Genevieve home after the adoption paperwork was signed, continuing to bond with her, and being her dad every day afterward was surreal and incredible. It still is. Looking back on the drama that surrounded those stressful days after her birth makes Aly and me even more thankful for her than if we'd had a child naturally and easily. I had seen God heal my wife, but that Monday morning in the hospital—when all hope was lost—was the first time I'd ever seen an unmistakable, real-time, instant miracle. God showed up in such an undeniable way, putting His stamp of approval on this adoption and making it clear to everyone involved that He had chosen *us* to be Genevieve's parents. It was a crazy situation—one we never expected but will never forget.

Afterward, as we were talking about everything that led to our having Genevieve, Aly remarked, "Our life should be a Lifetime movie!" We didn't realize at the time that television would indeed become a big part of our life . . . but that's a story for another chapter. For now, we were just focusing on getting used to life with our Genevieve.

POST-ADOPTION SYNDROME

Once we joined the ranks of parenthood, we got hit with the same question that people seem to ask every new mom and dad: "Do you guys want more children?" Why is this the first thing people ask you when you have a new baby? We always answered the same way, telling them that we wanted what God wanted for us—but we were perfectly content with one. That was the truth, and honestly, I wasn't sure if Aly could emotionally handle the challenges that would come with another adoption. This had been such a long, hard process full of the highest highs and lowest lows we could have imagined.

I think Aly's reaction to the "more kids" question was the same as any brand-new mom. If you ask a woman who's just given birth if she wants more kids, she'll probably tell you no. Or never. Or she might just say, "Are you crazy? Get away from me! Don't make me hurt you!" Seriously, whether it's an adoption or a traditional birth, that is such the wrong time to ask a mom if she wants more children!

—ALY—

I'd like to say Josh is exaggerating, but he's probably *underselling* what I felt during those first few months as a mom. As a therapist, I knew all the telltale signs of postpartum depression (PPD), and I know it can be a serious, draining, and painful experience for women. I'm not sure I'd go as far as to say I was in a full-blown PPD, but I was close. We had been through so much. We had moved our lives hundreds of miles away from home, created a lifelong relationship with Genevieve's birth family, almost lost her, experienced a miracle, and were now back home with a newborn as first-time parents. It was exhausting. I get why people ask about having more kids because there's such baby fever when you're around a newborn, but I wasn't in any kind of emotional place to even consider another adoption yet. I was going through what I started calling *post-adoption syndrome.*

Our journey connected us with countless other families who have adopted, and they all echoed what I was feeling. The worry and exhaustion that parents who adopt feel are identical to the stressors biological parents feel. Then, on top of that, there is a whole new set of issues that are unique in adoption scenarios. The biggest is the looming threat of adoption failure, which I can only compare to a miscarriage.

Please don't think I'm being insensitive to those who have walked through a miscarriage; my heart breaks for those families. While I haven't gone through the pain of having a miscarriage, I do know firsthand the pain of losing a child I'd already grown attached to. When Karen told us she was keeping Genevieve, it was as though we'd lost her forever. Then when God intervened, I felt like my child had come back to life. It sounds crazy, but that's the only way I can describe the ridiculous range of emotions I experienced. We were so blessed by our outcome, but I know many families who have experienced multiple adoption failures, and every one of them is devastating to a family expecting to bring a child home. I just didn't think I could risk going through that again.

Josh and I talked a lot about the state of our family during this time, and we ultimately agreed that having children—however God choses to give them—is not about *us* as parents. It's about the child, and it's about raising a boy or girl into a man or woman of God. I trusted God to work in and through me in a mighty way, but I was also aware of my capacity. Christian parents have an awesome responsibility to raise children to be disciples of Jesus Christ, and it's hard to admit, but I wasn't sure if I could do this with more than one child.

So, let's see. I was a cancer survivor who had beaten a life-threatening diagnosis, a new mom who had just been through an almost-failed adoption, and a woman in her twenties who had been told she was premenopausal and unable to have a child naturally without an egg donation. Mix that with the love I felt for my new baby girl, the stress I was under with my new parental responsibilities, and the sleepless nights every new parent goes through, and what do you get? You get a lady who clung to sanity only by screaming, "That's enough! Whatever else may or may not happen in the future, I choose to be content with the life God's given me!"

I didn't *need* any more children. I didn't *want* any more drama. All I wanted was a nice, quiet, boring, *normal* life with my husband and daughter. Josh and I finally felt like life was going to slow down a little bit, and we were looking forward to hunkering down with our little family and enjoying raising this wonderful little girl.

SWEET, SWEET SURRENDER

When Genevieve was about nine months old, I went to eat with a friend who was experiencing infertility and considering adoption. This has become part of my ministry life; it is a joy to pray with others who are wanting a family, considering adoption, or continuing to try to have a child naturally. This friend had a strong desire to conceive a child and was asking the question many potential moms ask: Could she truly love a child she adopted as much as a baby she carried for nine months?

I could only answer with the experience I had been through. I told her I had no desire to become pregnant now. I confessed that, at one time in my life, the need to get pregnant had become an all-consuming idol to me. But during and after Genevieve's adoption, that desire was gone. Not that it wouldn't be amazing to experience, and if God allowed it, we would be ecstatic. But we loved Genevieve so much; there's no way we ever could have loved her more if I *had* given birth to her myself. I explained that once your baby is in your arms, the love you feel isn't even in question. It's an experience, a blessing you can't understand until you walk through it. You just have to trust someone who's been there.

I could see the stress and skepticism in her face. It was hard not to shake her and say, "DO IT! It will be the best decision of your life! Why would you *not* want to adopt?" But then I put myself in her shoes and remembered having those same questions and thoughts just months before we had Genevieve. I realized I was looking into my own face as I looked at this woman. I knew God had changed my heart's desire through conversations with other mothers and families who had adopted, and now God had given me the chance to speak those same words of hope to this sweet, young friend.

Surrender is a beautiful thing. I had learned to surrender to God's plan for my family. My surrender didn't come as quickly as I'm sure God would have liked, but it did happen. Now it was up to my friend to surrender as well. When she left that day, I could tell she was still struggling. I thought, *If she only knew.* One day she might.

THE BIGGEST SURPRISE OF OUR LIFE

Despite our total surrender and peace with the life God had given us with Genevieve, other people kept coming up to us and saying they'd never stopped praying for us to conceive. I always wanted to respond, "You can stop praying now. We have our little girl, and we trust God to do whatever He wants with our future." I never actually said that, but I felt it. God had given us so much through my healing and our adoption. I was at a place in my life when I truly didn't feel the need to ask for more. I stopped praying to conceive once we had Genevieve, and I felt strongly that, if we did choose to grow our family later, it would be through adoption. That seemed like such a high honor to me by then. I had a new attitude about adoption, and I understood what the Bible means when it says we are children who have been adopted by our heavenly Father. I knew how much I loved Genevieve and got a glimpse of how much God must love me. Adoption was *it* for us.

That didn't stop others, though—especially my father-in-law, Terry. It seemed like any time we talked about fertility, he would say, "I know you'll get pregnant!" I can't tell you how many times he would talk about it or my mother-in-law, Renea, would say, "You know, Terry still prays and believes you'll get pregnant!" I would laugh and think to myself, *Naïve Mr. Terry. We were told it's impossible, and we have our miracle Genevieve. He really can stop praying and saying that!* But his faith never wavered, even after I stopped praying about it myself.

Just after Thanksgiving 2015, when Genevieve was nine months old, I started feeling sick. I'd had a flare-up of cellulitis in my arm, which is basically a painful skin infection. My arm swelled up like Popeye and turned bright red while my doctor tried to get it under control. This went on for about five days before the pain and irritation improved. The doctor warned me, though, that a side effect of cellulitis is flu-like symptoms. And man, did I get hit with flu-like symptoms! I felt terrible. I had no appetite, felt nauseous all the time, had weird body aches, and generally felt like garbage.

Two weeks into these symptoms, I was trying to soldier on and force myself to get better. I got up early one morning to exercise before work, but I felt especially sick and tired. I worked out anyway, and while washing my hands during a mid-workout bathroom break, I noticed an old home pregnancy test leftover from our fertility treatment days. I bought them in bulk back then (because I obsessively checked pretty much every day), and I had one test left. No point wasting the last one, right? So, on a whim, I decided to take it. I peed on the strip, set it aside on its package, and went back to finish my workout. I completely forgot about it.

After my workout, I showered and started getting ready for work. As I walked through the bathroom toward the closet, I saw the test sitting where

I'd left it. I laughed at myself for taking the test. Hadn't we been through enough of this? How many times did I need to see a negative pregnancy test? Besides, the doctors were very clear that nothing short of an egg donor would put a baby inside of me. I walked over to the test to throw it away, but then I saw something I'd never seen before: two lines. I stopped dead in my tracks, thinking, *Wait . . . what? That can't be right, can it? I mean, two lines would mean that I'm . . . I'm . . .*

I ran over to the trash and dug out the package to double check the instructions. There, plain as day, the package confirmed it: two lines means pregnant. *This is not happening*, I thought. *How can this be happening?* I was totally freaking out in the bathroom while Josh slept on the other side of the door. I didn't want to wake him up and tell him all this because I wasn't sure yet if I really believed it myself. Instead, I decided to let him sleep and do a little investigation before I said anything. However, just in case this turned out to be real, I wanted to do something special. So I decided to make a little video of myself in our living room.

The video is hilarious. I was such a mess. I wanted so badly to be excited, but I was confused and scared. I couldn't really believe this was happening, but it was still pretty amazing to see *two lines* for the first time in my life. After I finished the quick video, I texted my OB-GYN, who was also a good friend, and sent her a picture of the little pregnancy test. She told me to take some deep breaths and come in that morning for a blood test.

I walked into work that day and my coworker Katina came into my office. I think God sent her to me because she had adopted her first child and had two biological children after that. I had to spill my news through tears. She cried with me and supported me, and all I could think about was how scared I was and how this would affect my Genevieve. Plus, I was so confused. I had felt certain that if God were to grow our family again, it would be through adoption. And yet every part of me that once wanted to experience pregnancy came screaming back to life in an instant. I was thrilled to potentially be carrying a baby, but I was also terrified about getting too excited about what could still be a big mistake.

As my blood was taken that morning, I realized my heart had already connected to what that little pregnancy test said was growing in my body. But I tried not to let my mind go completely there yet. *Were my symptoms just from my arm infection, or were they really symptoms of pregnancy? Had I ignored my own body giving me signals?* I got more nervous and more excited with every thought.

Later that afternoon I received a text message from my doctor confirming the news the cheap pregnancy test had already told me: I was pregnant! That news came with a caution, however. Knowing my history, she suggested we keep it quiet until I could come in for an ultrasound. And I couldn't stop thinking about what the fertility doctor told us earlier about the high likelihood of miscarriage if I ever did manage to get pregnant. Yes, there were a lot of questions and a million risks. For right now, though, I was pregnant. I, Aly Taylor, breast cancer survivor and so-called *barren woman*, was pregnant.

—JOSH—

I'll never forget coming home from work on December 2, 2015. Aly was giddy. I'd seen that look on her face before; it's how she looks when she's excited about giving me a big surprise. We had just decorated the house for Christmas—Genevieve's first Christmas, no less—and Aly wanted me to sit on the couch so she could give me an early Christmas present. This was music to my ears. I love gifts, and surprises are the best. Aly handed me an envelope, and I had no idea what her gift might be. A new truck? A four-wheeler? Whatever it was, I figured she had written the big reveal into a corny poem I was supposed to read. I ripped open the envelope, knowing my wife was about to blow my mind with something awesome. I had no way of knowing just *how* awesome the surprise would be.

Instead of an original Aly Taylor love poem, I saw a Scripture passage written on the card. I knew this verse. It was the scripture that had been prayed over Aly many times, including at the send-off party we had before our first trip to Houston. It was Psalm 128 (NLT):

How joyful are those who fear the LORD—
     all who follow his ways!
You will enjoy the fruit of your labor.
     How joyful and prosperous you will be!
Your wife will be like a fruitful grapevine,
     flourishing within your home.
Your children will be like vigorous young olive trees
     as they sit around your table.
That is the LORD's blessing
     for those who fear him.
May the LORD continually bless you from Zion.
     May you see Jerusalem prosper as long as you live.
May you live to enjoy your grandchildren.
     May Israel have peace!

As I read that passage again—now with nine-month-old Genevieve in my amazing, cancer-free, completely healed wife's arms babbling and smiling—I felt a dam break in my mind. I was immediately flooded with all the memories of the past few years.

Throughout Aly's cancer, we determined to do just what this passage says: fear the Lord. We knew we had labored through pain and trusted God to protect Aly and give me wisdom and strength. I spent so many days and nights praying for my wife to be like a fruitful grapevine and for her to flourish in every way. We prayed that children would be like vigorous young olive trees around our table. We prayed for His blessings and that we would prosper as a family. We prayed for long lives and that we would live to enjoy our grandchildren.

Psalm 128 was important during Aly's cancer fight, but it was downright critical when we were told Aly could not have children. We prayed and prayed that God would intervene as we recited the words of the psalm over Aly. Then, when we made the decision to adopt, I struggled with whether adoption meant we had given up on God answering our prayer. It took a while for me to realize that adoption wasn't a sign that we had given up our faith; instead, it was a living symbol that we were going to follow God's lead on how He had chosen to grow our family. All these thoughts, prayers, and emotions came racing back front and center as I sat there reading this psalm again. But I couldn't for the life of me understand what Aly was trying to tell me.

I remember thinking for a half second, *Is she pregnant?* before forcing the thought out of my head. It wasn't possible, so I didn't even want to go there. The only other thing I could think of was that Aly had reached out to someone about adopting another baby. But that didn't make sense either, because there was no way she'd do that without talking to me. I was clueless. Finally, after I finished reading the passage and had a few moments to think through what was happening, Aly handed me another envelope. This one had a note with two words written at the top. It was two words I never thought I'd hear from my wife: *I'm pregnant!* Just to drive the point home, the only other words on the card were, *I'm not kidding!*

I lost it. Totally and completely. I was a sobbing pile of mush on our sofa beneath the glow of our Christmas lights. I could not wrap my head around what was happening or why it was happening now; I had a million questions. The only question I didn't ask was *how* it was happening. I knew how. The only thing I really knew for sure in that moment was that God had done it. He can and does do more than we could ever ask, hope, or imagine.

When Aly was diagnosed, God said, "Yeah, this is going to be hard. But trust Me. I got this." Later, when Aly's womb was closed, God said, "No worries. Genevieve needs a mom and a dad, and you guys need Genevieve." Then when Genevieve was ours, God said, "Oh yeah. Now it's time for Me to fulfill that *other* promise. You guys ready?"

And now Aly was pregnant! I know God can do anything and I'm sure He still has miracles in store for us, but I don't think I'll ever be more surprised or overwhelmed by the goodness of God than I was that night. The Christmas before we had learned we would have Genevieve, and now a year later, my wife was miraculously pregnant. Christmas miracles happening in our family is apparently a trend.

GUARDED BUT HOPEFUL

Aly's doctor wanted to see her soon because of her history. We walked into the appointment as excited as any expectant parents, but everyone else in the room was quiet and somber. It was as if everyone was afraid to be hopeful. Our hearts sank further when the doctor's expression grew even more somber. We had seen that look way too many times from way too many doctors, and we knew it wasn't good. The doctor explained that the little sac that is usually seen at this point in a new pregnancy was there, but there was nothing inside it. She went on to explain that it could be because Aly was too early in her pregnancy to see a yolk sac inside or it could be that a baby was not forming. Aly would need to come back in a few days for another ultrasound to see which of these scenarios was true.

So our first pregnancy appointment quickly went from hopeful excitement to disappointment and fear. I didn't feel good about the appointment at all. It's in my nature to protect Aly and myself, so I wanted to go with a "wait and see" attitude from the beginning. Aly, naturally, couldn't help but be excited. She wanted to believe she was carrying a little baby. But there was no mistaking the doctor's face. And that was enough for me to doubt that our baby was growing inside Aly. Her *I'm pregnant!* note was my highest mountaintop; the doctor's worried expression was the lowest valley. Once again there was nothing to do but wait and pray. Man, I was starting to really hate those words.

—ALY—

Josh and I were going crazy bouncing between excited and terrified, and we didn't want to take anyone else along for the ride. We'd already put our family through so much, and we didn't have the heart to get their hopes up until we got a better report from the doctor. So we kept our mouths shut—*mostly.* I had already told my friend at work, and I also reached out to a trusted friend who leads an infertility group. I needed her to pray with me about all this. We prayed over the phone, and she promised to keep praying for us as we waited for the next appointment. I have no doubt she kept her promise.

Isn't it funny how, when we're hurting, we rarely run to the person who seems to have it all together? Instead, we seek out those who have been through the same pain and fear we're experiencing, probably because we need to connect with someone who can relate to our particular challenges. I'm so grateful for others who have been through some of the same struggles. I needed it as I fought cancer, I needed it as I struggled through infertility, I needed it as we tried to navigate the adoption process, and now I needed it in the face of an uncertain pregnancy. I would never wish those kinds of troubles on anyone, but I'm so glad there are other women who have been through them. God blessed me so much with their wisdom and experience!

So, if you are struggling today and maybe even questioning the goodness of God, let me encourage you. Your trials and troubles are qualifying you to help someone else. There is someone out there who needs (or will need) your experience. God is so good to put people in our lives who have walked a similar path; and when we experience pain and hardship, we must choose to believe He is preparing us to be a blessing to others in the future. At that point in my life, maybe more than any other, I needed people to support me as I waited for my next doctor's appointment. My friend helped carry that burden with me when it seemed too heavy for me to bear alone.

—JOSH—

Guarded. That's how I can describe my attitude during that week of waiting. The morning of the appointment, though, Aly sat me down and told me she needed me to go into the appointment with a hopeful heart. We'd been down that road before when she told me she needed me to believe with her that she was healed, so I didn't even try to argue. I did my best to change my attitude. The best I could do was *guarded . . . but hopeful.*

We walked into the doctor's office, exchanged pleasantries with the staff we'd come to know, and then got to the business at hand: the ultrasound. They hooked up everything and we all held our breath. Immediately we could all tell the images looked much different from the week before. We could see something inside the sac; it was a baby! A beautiful, tiny, magnificent little Baby Taylor. We even heard the heartbeat! We were overjoyed, but our doctor, God bless her, still maintained her cautious optimism. Apparently she was *guarded but hopeful* too. She reminded us that there was still a high chance of complications, but that didn't matter at that moment. Finally, *finally . . .* Aly was carrying a baby.

As we were wrapping up, the doctor asked Aly if she wanted to come in every week for the next several weeks to check on things or if she wanted to handle this like any other pregnancy and only come in for regular visits. I expected Aly to take her up on her offer, especially after we'd been given so many warnings about so many possible problems. However, Aly told her she wanted to approach it as a normal pregnancy. This was another *wow* moment for me. I'm continually humbled and astounded by my wife's amazing faith. Seeing her boldness and unflinching confidence that God would take care of her knocked my guard down. From that point on, I was only *hopeful*.

PRAYERS OF THE FAITHFUL

Aly and I had a blast telling our family and friends the good news. Watching the reality sink in—seeing them first assume we were adopting a second child and then finally realizing we were pregnant—was the best feeling in the world. After sharing so much bad news over the years, it was wonderful to celebrate this new miracle with them. As we told more and more people, we were surprised to hear so many friends tell us the exact same thing. In their own way, many of them said, "You know, we never actually *stopped* praying for you guys to get pregnant, even after you had Genevieve. We've been praying for this for years now." We later learned that hundreds of others who followed our story on the blog had been doing the exact same thing. God had answered the prayers of His faithful.

—ALY—

I used to think God meets us at our level of faith. I often believed the enemy's lies, thinking that if I just believed more, did more, or prayed more, things would go differently for me. But that mind-set can be a trap. It puts all the work (and hope) solely on *me*. That mentality takes away my dependence on the Lord and makes me feel as though I have power over life and death myself. Yes, I know I have free will and the power to choose to walk out God's plan for my life. I also know that many of God's promises come with conditions. But believing in God means knowing *I* am not the healer. *I* am not the difference maker. *I* am not the final word.

Can I follow God's purpose and plan for my life? Yes. Can I experience His promises in fullness if I obey and submit to Him? Yes. But can I, with all my best efforts, miraculously change my situation without God doing the work Himself? No. Trying to meticulously craft my future only leaves me tired, frustrated, and doubting God.

I was amazed to realize that, even though I had stopped praying to conceive, my situation changed because others had not. I became pregnant because God answered my father-in-law's prayers. He answered my family's prayers. He answered the prayers that were lifted up by a circle of friends the night before we first left for Houston. He answered the prayers of hundreds of strangers who only knew Josh and me through our blog. I was pregnant not because I had prayed or done anything miraculous; I was pregnant because God *made* me pregnant, and because other people's prayers were in agreement with His perfect will for my life.

I say all this with much thanksgiving and humble gratitude. I know there are millions of people who pray for pregnancy who never get pregnant. There are millions of people who pray for healing who are never healed this side of heaven. Does that mean my prayers were special or that God chose to bless us instead of someone else? Absolutely not! Our prayers just happened to align with His will for us to be blessed with a child.

If you're reading this and still waiting for God to work a miracle, trust that He is in the process of working out His will for your life. If you're trying to get pregnant, trust Him to add a baby *if*, *how*, and *when* He sees fit. If you are praying for healing, trust God in this season of suffering and believe that He is somehow going to make it all work together for your good. Through all our struggles, I've had to learn to pray not for what Josh and I want, but for God to accomplish His will in our lives. That's often meant asking God to make *us* passionate about what *He's* passionate about—even if it's something that's not even on our radar.

I've also learned to pray by believing and speaking scripture over my requests. That way I know every part of my life has been covered with God's

Word and prayer and total belief that He is sovereign in my life. Whether His answer is yes, no, or wait, I can rest in knowing I have trusted Him and put my life in His hands.

So, yes, this pregnancy was an unexpected miracle. A baby of faith. A surprise. A joy. I thought He would have us expand our family again through adoption, but apparently He had other plans . . . or did He? What we couldn't have guessed then was that God had another miraculous surprise for us. Believe it or not, our lives were about to get even crazier.

CHAPTER 10

SHE CHOSE US . . . AGAIN

—JOSH—

It took a little while, but Aly and I finally wrapped our heads around the fact that she was pregnant and that we were about to be a family of four. Having two kids so close in age can be a challenge, but under those circumstances, it was even more shocking for us. As Aly got past her initial pregnancy sickness and started feeling better, our "Houston family," the Stanfills, invited me on a hunting trip in South Texas at their camp. Aly gave me the green light (probably because she knew it'd be much harder for me to get away after we had two kids), and I was soon heading off to Texas for a little fun.

Somewhere along the way during my thirteen-hour drive, I got a phone call that almost made me drive off the road in shock. I saw a number flash on my phone and noticed it was the attorney we used for our adoption. We hadn't talked to him in a while, but we were still paying some bills from the adoption, so I figured he needed to let me know about a new processing fee, filing fee, or another one of the million fees that had popped up since we brought Genevieve home. When I answered, however, I quickly realized this call had nothing to do with our payment plan. I sat there stunned as the attorney gave me some news I never would have imagined in a thousand years. Our lives were about to change forever. Again.

THE CALL HEARD AROUND THE WORLD

—ALY—

I was a little nervous about being a solo mom with Genevieve for the weekend, especially since I'd felt so sick for the past few weeks. However, I was glad Josh had the opportunity to get away, and I thought it'd be a good chance for me to get some rest too. My plan was simple: sleep whenever Genevieve slept. It's every new mom's dream, but it rarely works out. This day was no different.

Genevieve had just gone down for her afternoon nap, and I was ready for a little doze myself. Before collapsing onto the sofa, I checked my phone and noticed a missed call from a number I didn't recognize. I listened to my voicemail and was pleased to hear a message from Genevieve's birth grandmother. We hadn't talked to her since we left the hospital that incredible Monday morning nine months earlier, so I called her back to catch up.

We slid right into our old comfort level as we chatted. I told her all about Genevieve, and we marveled together at how she was going to be a big sister. It was great to hear from her, but I could tell she was a little nervous and wanted to discuss something important. I couldn't guess what bomb she was about to drop.

When I asked how Karen was doing, she told me Karen was pregnant again. I wasn't sure what to say; the way she said it definitely didn't make it sound like *good* news. My hope and prayer for Genevieve's birth mom was always that she'd one day be in a place to have a family of her own, but that didn't seem to be what her mother was telling me. She went on to explain that Karen was really struggling and, once again, knew she wouldn't be able to care for a baby. Then she asked, "Would you two be open to adopting again?"

I was absolutely speechless. She said she felt silly asking, especially now that she knew I was eight weeks pregnant. However, she and Karen felt strongly that we would be their first choice to adopt this new baby. Everything in me wanted to scream, "Yes! Yes, of course we will!" I already felt such a strong connection to this baby, even though I didn't know anything about him or her. Karen hadn't been to the doctor yet, so they didn't even know the due date. It was January, and they assumed the baby would arrive early summer. I was due in August, just a couple of months later.

My head was spinning. I thanked her for calling, told her I loved her, and said I'd talk it over with Josh and get back to her. As soon as I hung up, I fell on my knees and asked God for wisdom in how to talk to Josh about all this. I could already tell where my heart was leaning, but how could I put all this on my husband after we'd been through so much already?

Little did I know Josh had already received the same news I had. We had a lot to talk about.

—JOSH—

I couldn't believe what the attorney told me. Karen was pregnant again? And she wanted us to adopt this baby too? My first thought—my *only* thought—was, *Yes! Absolutely!* That may sound crazy, especially since I had a nine-month-old and my wife was pregnant. But the thought of having *another* Genevieve under any circumstance was a no-brainer for me. I was *in*, but I had no idea what Aly would say. Genevieve was practically still a newborn to us, and we had *just* gotten used to the idea that we were pregnant. What if she and I were on different pages about this opportunity? I resisted the urge to call Aly to tell her the news and decided to pray the rest of the way to Rocksprings, Texas. I really wanted to have my thoughts together before we talked about it. About ten seconds later, my phone rang. It was Aly. I answered, hoping I'd be able to keep my mouth shut about the attorney's call.

Aly immediately launched into the details of her call with Karen's mother. When we each realized the other already knew the situation, I took a breath and asked Aly what she was thinking. "I think I want to do it," she said. "But we can't jump into it. We've got to pray about it, talk more with the birth family and attorney, and make sure all this is *really* real." I just love that about my wife. She was scared and exhausted, but her first thought was to pray about how we could make this work. That was a huge step for anyone, but especially a new mom who had just been through one adoption and was in the middle of her own first trimester. We had learned firsthand that adoption is an amazing experience, but it is an emotional whirlwind. We had to be certain we were ready to jump back into the storm.

—ALY—

It surprised me a little bit that Josh and I both already felt an instant connection to this new baby, but it really shouldn't have. We had already prayed about this child a lot, even though we didn't know *this* was the child we were praying for. After Genevieve was born, we were content to have this one perfect little girl, though we would have loved for her to have siblings. However, the adoption process had been challenging, so I prayed, *Lord, if You want us to adopt again, please don't make us go through an agency and deal with the whole process from scratch. If it's something You want us to do, make it plain and clear and something we don't even have to apply for.*

When I prayed those words, I was thinking the next opportunity would come five or ten years later—not *nine months* later. I envisioned getting a call about a baby who'd been abandoned at the hospital and needed a home. But God was doing something even crazier. He was answering our prayer with an astounding yes, and He was giving Genevieve something precious: a sibling with her own shared DNA. The timing was not what we would have chosen, but this was clearly God answering our prayers once again.

—JOSH—

I spent that entire hunting trip consumed in thought and prayer about this situation. I kept praying for God to reveal His next step to me, and all I heard in response was, "Yes, yes, yes." I had no idea what I would do if Aly felt differently. There were so many unknowns. We didn't know the due date. We didn't know the gender—of this baby *or* the one Aly was carrying, for that matter. We didn't know how we'd handle three kids all under eighteen months at one time. But all I heard from God was a big, fat yes. I just couldn't imagine saying no to this opportunity.

When I finally got home from the longest weekend hunting trip in history, Aly and I just looked at each other. I think both of us knew what our decision would be. I told her what I was thinking, she told me what she was thinking, and that was it. We were all in. As we hugged and celebrated, she looked up at me and said, "Are we absolutely crazy?"

"Yes. Yes, we are," I replied. "But I don't care."

—ALY—

Crazy or not, here we come! We contacted the attorney and birth family to let them know we would love to adopt this baby and to get the process started. From there, all we could do for a while was trust God with the baby I was carrying and the one Karen was carrying too. Not long after, we discovered I was carrying another girl. We were thrilled that Genevieve would have a sister! We also learned that Karen was due later than we'd assumed. We originally thought the two babies would arrive a couple of months apart; however, our world was rocked again when we learned Karen's and my due dates were only three *weeks* apart. So, in a weird way, we were having twins!

THANK HEAVEN FOR LITTLE GIRLS

By this point, we were communicating regularly with Karen and her family, and we asked if she would allow us to come to one of her doctor visits to learn the gender of our other baby. She was so kind to allow us to do that. Karen had moved to Kentucky, so we packed up and made the drive north.

If you pictured the funny looks we got from people during our pedicure when she was pregnant with Genevieve, you should have seen us now! You can only imagine the questions and glances we received when we were at the ultrasound together, both obviously pregnant, explaining to the ultrasound technicians the nature of our relationship. My poor husband! He literally spent the day describing how and why he was the father of babies from two women! People were always amazed, but we had gotten used to it; it's just what our family is. It may not be *normal*, but most miracles aren't. That's what makes them miracles!

We learned in that ultrasound that we were having another little girl. *Three baby girls!* Genevieve would be just seventeen months old when her sisters were born, and we knew our lives were going to be turned upside down in the best way possible.

After that appointment, we went back home to get things ready. I loved feeling my baby growing inside me; every little movement was a testament that she was strong and healthy. It was a struggle not having that same assurance with our other baby. We had no control over Karen's prenatal care or what activities she was doing. We trusted her, of course, but it was hard being responsible for the health of only one of my baby daughters. All I could do is trust and pray—so I prayed like a mad woman!

—JOSH—

Three little girls. I was ecstatic! I can honestly say I never really hoped for a boy. I might have hoped for one before infertility or before we experienced the unbelievable blessing of a daughter, but I didn't care at this point. I was mainly thankful for a houseful of babies, and the fact that we were adding two more little girls after I'd spent the past year loving Genevieve like crazy was icing on the cake. Sure, people joked about three weddings, three college students, and three times the drama, but I wasn't worried. Those were all bridges we'd cross later. I was more concerned with raising three ladies of strong, godly character. I knew I could handle any errant hormone battles that were in our future. That's a small price to pay for the honor of raising three powerful women of faith and launching them into the world to do amazing things for the kingdom of heaven.

—ALY—

Naming these little ladies was an awesome responsibility. I knew from years of Bible study that names are extremely important in Scripture. Sometimes a child is born and the passage itself tells you what the chosen name means. Other times God actually renames someone as a way of redirecting his or her entire life. So, as I considered each name, I spent hours praying over the name and its meaning. I poured through Scripture looking for strong women of faith, and I looked through countless books, searching for names that reflected the meaning we wanted to convey. I wanted the names we chose to be powerful and meaningful. I wanted their names to speak prophetically over their lives. We felt like we were blessed with inspiration when we named Genevieve Rose, and we wanted our other two girls to have that same blessing.

We chose the name *Vera* for the girl I was carrying. Vera means "faith," and we believed wholeheartedly that this was our faith baby. She was the child we were told was impossible, but she was *made* possible by faith. We prayed that she would rest in her faith in Christ and always have faith in God's great might and power as she faces the adversities in her life.

Then we chose the name *Lydia* for the baby we were adopting. I kept coming back to this name over and over as we prayed. It's a beautiful name, and I loved its meaning: "woman of God." When I think of all the things I want our girls to be, "woman of God" encompasses it all! With the names set, we prayed every day for our three beautiful daughters by name, asking God to lead, guide, and protect them all the days of their lives.

DELIVERY DILEMMA

As my pregnancy went on, I started getting nervous about how close the two due dates were. I became afraid that I'd miss Lydia's birth. If Vera came a little late and Lydia came a little early, there'd be no way I could make the journey from Louisiana to Kentucky in time to be in the delivery room to see Lydia enter the world. That experience meant everything to me when Genevieve was born, and the thought of not having that same immediate, day-one connection with Lydia became a huge stressor for me.

One of the big issues was travel. The best-case scenario was that I'd have to travel out of state with a newborn almost immediately after giving birth. And then there was the question of where we'd stay in Kentucky. Fortunately, my awesome husband came to the rescue. Josh was discussing all these concerns with a friend and he replied, "Hey, Josh. Why don't you guys take our motor home to Kentucky? You can stay in it while you're there getting Lydia." This was such a blessing to us, and it took some of the pressure off. At least now we knew where we'd stay. But there was still the issue of timing.

I had a wonderful relationship with my OB-GYN and was excited for her to deliver Vera. She had been with us through the whole infertility ordeal, so she knew how much of a miracle Vera was. We had spent time developing our birth plan—natural childbirth with no epidural— and she was supportive of every one of our decisions. However, it dawned on me that everything would have to go perfectly with both pregnancies and both babies would have to arrive very close to their due dates in order for us to be present for Lydia's birth. Then it hit me: What if I had Vera in Kentucky? It would mean my doctor couldn't deliver her, but that one decision would put every one of my other fears to rest. We would be closer to the birth mother, we'd be able to participate in her last few weeks of pregnancy, and we'd almost certainly be able to be there for Lydia's birth.

It felt a little crazy to leave our home, doctor, and support system right before giving birth, but I really thought this was the answer. When I explained my idea to Josh, he agreed right away. That's one of the things I love most about Josh: he never finds my ideas crazy or ridiculous. Because he's a radical, outside-the-box thinker himself, he never tries to talk me down from an idea. Instead, he encourages it and sometimes even adds new ideas to it. They don't all work out, but it's a huge blessing to have such a great partner with me on this grand adventure.

—JOSH—

We went into deep research mode, trying to find the right doctor and hospital for Aly in Kentucky. Many doctors won't take new pregnancies after the thirty-six-week mark, so we had to do some digging. We finally found a place that would take her. She'd be cared for by a midwife and deliver Vera at a wonderful hospital in Indiana just over the Kentucky state line. The plan was set. We would do the following:

- Drive my thirty-six-week pregnant wife, sixteen-month-old baby, and myself to a motor park in Kentucky, where we'd live huddled up in a borrowed motor home for a month.
- Change all Aly's doctors and caregivers in the last few weeks of her pregnancy.
- Deliver our miracle baby in a hospital we'd never seen with a midwife we hadn't met yet.
- Have one baby in time to be in the delivery room for the other.

- Finalize new adoption papers and processes.
- Come home a month later as a family of five.

Sounds simple enough, right?

Oh, and to keep things interesting, I should also mention that right before we headed to Kentucky, I lost my job. Aly had recently left her school counseling job to be home with our now growing family, and my job loss added much financial unknowns and stress. Talk about perfect timing. Thankfully, I had a side job that would help with some provision. Aly and I were devastated and more than a little concerned about what we'd do, but we knew God would provide; He always had. Besides, we knew the next month would be enough to handle without us worrying about getting back to punch a time clock.

—ALY—

Josh losing his job hit us hard. It may be easy to read our story and assume the only stressors in our lives were cancer, infertility, adoption, and now figuring out this new birth plan. Sure, those were life-changers, but we still had all the same problems and concerns as everyone else. Finances, in particular, were a struggle, especially considering all the medical bills, then the fertility treatments, and then the adoption fees. The thought of going through the next month and then getting home with five mouths to feed and no dependable, predictable income was terrifying.

It would be easy for me to go off on a huge tangent right now about how incredible Josh is, what a wonderful provider he's always been, and how God continued to care for us in the face of this job loss, but those things are a little beyond the scope of this book. I will, however, share an excerpt here from a blog post I wrote while processing the unknowns while we were in the motor home in Kentucky. It captures where we were faithwise in the middle of our lives taking such a dramatic turn.

July 20, 2016

So, here we are, trusting God has gone before us. We are taking this time in Kentucky to pray about Josh's future employment and that he does exactly what God would have him do. Josh is a powerhouse and a workhorse. I am not a wife who worries if he finds something to do. I am not worried he will be lazy or that we won't have an income. We have no doubt he will find something else to do.

We are more concerned about him taking a job that is God's will and not just jumping on the first thing that comes his way. And that can be easy to do and pressure-filled when you are having two new babies coming into our family in the coming days/weeks. . . .

Even though, from a worldly perspective, it seems like the timing of all this couldn't be worse, we have seen God do too many things in our life to not trust that His timing is perfect.

What circumstance are you currently allowing to dampen or dilute your faith? Were you at one point extremely passionate and faithful about something in your life, and because of circumstances you allowed that faith to be dug up and replaced with doubt? Please join us and do not let this happen! Let's be a force together! From two people who are currently battling with this daily, join us! We know that God is holding us in His hands, and we can trust Him.

You can too.

I fully believe that we will be able to share very soon how God has led us to something that is amazing. Just pray that we follow God's leading and continue to trust the God who has NEVER let us down.

When I wrote that, I knew God had bigger and better things in store for us. I just didn't know how public that new plan would be. But I was about to find out.

CHAPTER 11

KENTUCKY BOUND

—ALY—

Smack-dab in the middle of the craziest summer of our lives—thirty-six weeks pregnant and about to head to Kentucky to give birth to one girl and adopt another—God surprised us once again. Up to this point, we had been pretty public about our story and had shared openly (and vulnerably) on the blog and in our speaking engagements. We had given hundreds of followers access to the highs and lows of our cancer battle, adoption experience, and now our pregnancy. We never did that for our own fame and attention; the goal from the start was to provide a platform for us to glorify God with our journey and to ask for specific prayers along the way. We expected Him to do miracles, and we wanted to encourage others with what He was doing in our lives. So from day one we tried to make Him the focus of every blog post and every speaking opportunity we had. Little did we realize what He had in store for us.

Right before we left for Kentucky, we were contacted by a production company who worked for TLC television network. They were planning the second season of their show *Rattled*, and they asked if we wanted to participate. *Rattled* is a reality show that follows several families through pregnancy and the first year or so of parenthood. If you have kids, you know why *Rattled* is such a great name for this show! Our involvement would mean we'd have film crews following us around, interviewing us, and getting a front-row seat into our real, unedited, and often messy lives. And, of course, they wanted to start immediately, meaning they'd be there for Vera's birth and for Lydia's adoption process in Kentucky.

I'm sure a lot of people would have been thrilled to get this phone call, but my first—and strongest—reaction was a definitive *heck no*. I thought, *There is no way I want to have my kids on TV*. It would have been so easy to cut off the conversation right there. But God wouldn't leave me alone about it.

Josh and I talked through it, got some advice from godly mentors, and prayed over the decision. Once the shock and intimidation wore off a little, we started to see how God could use this opportunity. We realized we would be able to share our miracle story with a national audience and, in turn, give many people hope. I worked hard to take the focus off myself and kids and put it back where we'd tried to keep it all along: on God. What could He do with this show? How many people would He encourage through our story? TLC said they at least wanted to document us living in Kentucky, Vera's birth, and Lydia's adoption. They assured us Lydia's birth family would have complete privacy, and they agreed to let us share the bigger picture of our family, faith and all. With those assurances in place, we agreed to live our lives on TV for a few months.

Knowing God had given us a bigger platform to share His goodness, we had three specific prayers for the show. First, we prayed that people going through cancer would be given hope. We wanted to show cancer patients that there is victory and new life on the other side of the fight. Second, we prayed that people facing infertility would be encouraged. To see us go from "infertile" to running around crazy with three babies would definitely be a cause for hope! Third, we wanted to shine a spotlight on the beauty of adoption so that any viewers who were on the fence about adopting would commit to giving a child a home. We knew that God answers prayer, so we were excited to see what He would do with this unexpected opportunity.

So that's what July 2016 looked like for us. We had a sixteen-month-old running around, I was thirty-six weeks pregnant, we were going to adopt another newborn within days of me delivering, I had quit my job only months before Josh learned he lost his main employment, and we were all going to live crammed inside a motor home out of state and away from our support system during the most stressful, demanding month of our lives. Oh, and a film crew was going to be in our faces capturing most every laugh, tear, conversation, and argument we had throughout the whole ordeal. You're probably thinking, *They must be crazy.* Well . . . you're right. It was nuts, but it was our life!

RATTLED—FOR REAL

—JOSH—

We thought we'd have a little time to adjust in Kentucky before the film crew showed up. Wrong. When we drove into the motor home park after a long drive from Louisiana, we found a team of producers and cameramen waiting on us. They were on us from the second we stepped foot on Kentucky soil. Aly and I looked at each other, thinking, *What on earth have we signed up for?* It was a reality check for us. We were already feeling homesick and worried about what life would be like with cameras following us around 24-7. We had to stop and remind ourselves that God had put this whole crazy situation into motion. We were about to have three amazing, miraculous little girls, and He would get all the glory. It was pretty humbling.

We spent a couple of days getting settled in the RV park and doing our first round of interviews for *Rattled*, and then Aly had her first checkup with her new midwife. If there was ever any doubt about the care we'd receive in Kentucky, it vanished as soon as we met the midwife. She was awesome. She immediately put Aly at ease, and I could tell the two of them hit it off right from the start. She explained that she likes to do everything naturally, but Aly would deliver in a hospital so she could call in a medical team if something unexpected happened. As an added bonus, this hospital was full of believers. That meant we would be surrounded by people who loved Jesus and were praying for us. They knew how much of a miracle this baby was.

Meanwhile, as we were getting Aly settled with her new medical team, we were able to join Lydia's birth mother for her doctor appointments too. Karen's father came with her to many of these appointments, and it was great being able to get to know him better. Things were so different this time around because we already had a relationship with Karen; we had a year and a half of history together. The last time I'm sure Karen worried about how we'd raise Genevieve, but now she had seen how much we adored our daughter. In fact, she commented several times that it felt like Aly had given birth to Genevieve herself. All that made her fully trust us this time, and I know it took a lot of pressure off her. Plus, it made all of us a lot more comfortable together in these final weeks before the girls were born.

I can't describe how beautiful it was watching Aly and Karen go through doctor appointments and ultrasounds together. They laughed together, cried together, and enjoyed telling each other stories. As untraditional as it was, this was *our family*, and it was a joy to spend those weeks with Karen and her family. At one point, however, she gave us a big scare. Aly was only a week from her own due date when Karen called us to tell us she was heading to the hospital with strong contractions. We rushed to the hospital, not sure what we'd find, but it turned out to be false labor. She was in a lot of pain, though. We helped calm her down, prayed for her, and let her know how much we loved her. The doctor sent her home, and Aly and I thanked God for putting us so close to her during those tense weeks.

—ALY—

My appointments were getting a little worrisome too. After every doctor visit, we thought Vera would arrive any minute. I was dilated and effaced, and the midwife kept telling us we were almost ready. My mom and Josh's mom joined us in Kentucky as my due date neared; they didn't want to risk missing anything! Everything was progressing perfectly as we counted down the days. Then the big day finally arrived—and nothing happened. Then Vera was one day late. Then two. Then three. Finally, three days after the due date, I woke up in the middle of the night with strong contractions. I called my doula (or birth coach) and thought it was time, but the contractions settled down, and I fell back to sleep. I went to the midwife the next day and she said everything looked fine, but I still wasn't in labor.

We started getting worried about Vera being so late and Lydia possibly coming early. I had this nightmare scenario in my head of Karen and me going into labor at the exact same minute. Every day I didn't go into labor brought us one day closer to Karen going into labor. I was trying so hard not to become too anxious, but it was nerve-racking. It didn't help that I was *really* uncomfortable. I was five centimeters dilated but still not in active labor. Come on! My big prayer had been to have Vera on time so that I could enjoy that experience and soak up a week or two with her before Lydia came along, but now there was a real chance that wouldn't happen.

Karen and I were in constant contact; we texted each other about different symptoms and how we were feeling. I occasionally had "pinch me" moments when it suddenly occurred to me who I was talking to and what I was talking about. It was definitely not your typical birth *or* adoption scenario.

Josh and I decided we needed a backup plan just in case Karen and I went into labor at the same time. I desperately wanted to be there for Lydia's birth, but that was starting to look iffy—especially since Karen and I were delivering at different hospitals. After discussing various options, I finally looked at Josh and said, "If we are in labor at the same time, I want you to go with her." He really struggled with this; after everything we'd been through, it crushed us both to imagine him *not* being in the delivery room with me when our miracle baby was born. However, the reality was that Lydia would need him too. I'd have our mothers in the room supporting me, but it was important to me that at least one of us be there for Lydia from the moment she entered the world. After discussing it a little more, we eventually decided this was our backup plan. But we still prayed like crazy it wouldn't come to that.

A SURPRISE REACTION

By August 13, I was four days late and getting frustrated. Fortunately, I was surrounded by my favorite people. My sister, Jessica, had driven in to surprise me, our "Houston mom," Tammy, was there, and, of course, our parents were still hanging around waiting on our baby girls. Everyone had found their own place to stay, mostly in basement apartments or friends-of-friends' homes. Eventually, though, we decided to look for one place that would house us all. We found a great home to rent for a few weeks that would enable all of us to be under one roof amid all this craziness. That was such a blessing! Once again God gave us the perfect place to stay at the perfect time.

Finally, I started feeling contractions. They weren't regular; they just came on here and there. I used my phone to track them and decided to stay active to speed things along. We ate lunch and took a long walk downtown. Then we went to the mall to walk. Just picture all of us—the whole family—power walking around a mall trying to convince Vera to come out and meet everyone. It was a sight! The contractions sped up and felt more consistent, so we decided to head to the hospital to see if this was the real deal. I still wasn't completely certain, but I sure didn't want to have my baby in the middle of the mall! At the hospital the midwife confirmed that I was in active labor and had dilated to six centimeters. This was it—another Taylor baby was about to make her appearance!

It's important to remember that we had film crews following us around for all of this. They got every dramatic second of it on tape. It was weird having them there for such private moments, but I did my best to mentally block them out. I reminded myself how glad we'd be later to have all this so well-documented. That helped, but man . . . the thought of having all these people see me in so much pain and about to push out a baby was downright strange.

After more laps around the hospital, I became too uncomfortable to keep walking. I was in a lot of pain and just wanted to lie down. As they connected me to the monitors and an IV, they reminded me I had tested positive for Group B strep at a previous appointment, which is a common bacteria in pregnant women. It wasn't serious, but they had to give me an antibiotic to make sure the bacteria wasn't passed to Vera in the birth canal. Thankfully, my doula was there with the fan right by my sweaty face and encouraging me as they administered the antibiotic. As a side note: having both a doula and a midwife as part of my birth plan was an excellent choice for me. Each person is unique in what she needs during pregnancy and delivery and there are a lot of options out there. Go with what works for you—don't let anyone else's opinion weigh too heavily in what you want and need for yourself.

I knew labor was just beginning, but it was already more painful than I'd expected. Plus, as the antibiotic went into my system, I noticed that my face was swelling up. Honestly, my face felt like a water balloon, really tight and full and like it was about to burst. I mentioned this to my doula while fighting through a contraction, and she said it was probably just because I was tightening up so much from the pain of the contraction. She told me to do my best to relax my face as the contractions hit. I tried (as well as I could while also feeling the worst pain of my life), but my face kept feeling worse and worse. I thought it was going to explode from all the pressure.

At that point, I saw a frightened look on her face and the whole room went eerily silent. The doula rushed out of the room calling for the midwife. I heard people scurrying around the room, but it was getting harder for me to see. Something was wrong. The midwife came in and explained that the pressure I was feeling was definitely not normal. I was having a severe allergic reaction to the antibiotic they had pushed into my system, and it had caused my face to swell up like a balloon. I couldn't see at all now; my eyes had literally swollen shut. I had to rely on everyone to tell me who was in the room and what was happening.

The midwife assured me that I was going to be fine, and they stopped the antibiotic and were controlling the reaction with Benadryl. Of course, they couldn't give me the same dose of Benadryl they'd normally give someone in my condition, because, let's not forget, I was in active labor! They had to make sure I was awake and lucid enough to push when the time came. I couldn't believe this was happening. *Seriously?* Lying there miserable, in pain, swollen, frustrated, and blind, I tried to find *some* bright spot in all this. Then it hit me: *Hey, at least I can't see the camera crew filming me anymore!*

—JOSH—

Looking back, I can see how the scene could seem a little funny, but it was scary in the moment. I wasn't in the room when Aly first started reacting to the antibiotic, but I was in the hall when they came running out for the midwife. Getting all the way through nine months of pregnancy was already such a miracle for us. Seeing the doctors and nurses jump into action on an emergency call to my wife's delivery room was terrifying. I ran to Aly's room and quickly got up to speed on what was happening.

I'd like to say Aly was exaggerating about being swollen like a balloon . . . but I can't. It looked bad. Really, really bad. And it didn't help that she was in so much pain from the labor. Between contractions she talked about how much her face hurt; then a contraction would hit with such ferocity that she forgot all about her face and could only think about the pain in her stomach. When the contraction was over, her attention went back to her face. The poor girl couldn't get a break. Before the allergic reaction, the doula and nurses told her to take advantage of those wonderful little breaks between contractions, but she couldn't. She was stuck in a horrible cycle of stomach pain, face pain, stomach pain, face pain, stomach pain, face pain. I was so grateful Karen wasn't also in labor, because I couldn't imagine not being there for Aly during all this.

MEETING VERA

—ALY—

Nothing could have prepared me for what I was going through. It all seemed surreal, and I could not make sense of what was happening around me. At one point someone came into the room, stood next to me, and said a sweet prayer for me. When she was finished, I said, "Uh . . . who are you?"

She replied, "It's Renea. You know, your *mother-in-law*." I couldn't see anything or anyone, and I had a loud electronic fan blowing in my face so I couldn't hear well either. Everyone had a great laugh at me not recognizing the voice of a woman I'd known more than half my life! I didn't find it *quite* as funny at the time, though.

I had made such great plans for this miraculous birth, but nothing was working out the way I thought it would. I wanted to labor in the bath tub, but there was a citywide water ban the night I was in the hospital. I wanted to have praise and worship music playing in the background while I was in labor, but the film crew said we couldn't have music on. I wanted Josh to read scripture cards to me that I had personally made in advance. Okay, this one we actually *did* get to do . . . but it was seriously the most annoying thing I had ever heard in my life. Sorry, Jesus! It was me, not You! It's so funny how we try to plan out all the key moments of our lives, but when the time comes, we find we have almost no control over anything. All we can do is pray that God's will would be done.

Soon the contractions got unbearable and I couldn't imagine going through this for one more second. I felt a lot of pressure like I needed to push, and the midwife told me I was ready; it was time to push my baby out.

The nurse described all the different positions I could use to deliver the baby. I always pictured myself on my back with my legs pulled up; I had no idea there were so many options. One of the positions she mentioned was basically on all fours, facedown with my hands and knees on the table. For some reason that position sounded like the most comfortable, so we went with it. Mind you, with my eyes sealed shut and my body overwhelmed with pain, I had completely forgotten about the TV cameras. So there I was: a water-balloon face, swollen eyes, crippling pain, and crouching on all fours trying to push out a baby—perfectly preserved on film for all of America to enjoy at their leisure. At that moment, though, I couldn't have cared less. All I wanted was to deliver the baby and for this madness to stop.

Finally, I pushed with everything I had in me and let out a scream I couldn't muster up again if I tried. And then . . . *relief.* I experienced the purest moment of relief and thankfulness of my life. It was done. They helped me roll over and lie on my back just in time for them to put the sweetest baby on my chest. Here she was, the baby everyone said couldn't happen. The child several doctors told me I'd never meet. The living miracle we could see, hear, and touch. I just kept thanking God over and over again as Josh and I wept. She was here. God made the impossible possible, and Vera Alyce Taylor was here.

—JOSH—

I was overcome with emotion the instant Vera appeared. Everything came full circle in that moment as I watched a strong, healthy, vibrant woman give birth to a beautiful, problem-free, full-term baby. I had seen Aly so sick and weak over the past several years. We had even had a couple of conversations about her funeral during some especially bad times. But those days were gone. Here she was, happy and cancer-free, bringing our daughter into the world. Psalm 128 was made manifest in my life, and the moment completely undid me.

Standing there with Aly and Vera in my arms, I wept in thankfulness to God. I don't even know what I said. I just felt His Spirit pouring out of me in a way I'd only felt one other time—when I prayed in the hospital with Karen after we thought Genevieve wouldn't be ours. I guess the Holy Spirit just takes over for me when I'm overwhelmed with emotion for my wife, children, and God's goodness to us. After the journey we'd been on, I knew it would be impossible for me to ever love my God or my family more.

Vera was born at 4:22 a.m. after an intense night of labor. When we had a minute to catch our breath, Aly checked her phone to see if we had missed any messages from Karen. Nothing! Thank God we didn't miss Lydia's birth and I didn't have to rush off to another hospital. I could focus on Aly and Vera for a while.

There are always some concerns when you bring a second child home for the first time. We knew Genevieve was a dream little girl, but we couldn't help but wonder how she'd react to this new baby in the house. We also weren't sure what she'd think when we brought *another* baby home a couple of weeks later. We didn't need to worry. From the instant we walked in the house with Vera, Genevieve was in love with her little sister. There was never even a hint of jealousy. Instead, Genevieve wanted to hold, kiss, and love on Vera all the time. She called the baby "Ra-Ra" and was totally obsessed with her. We all were.

ANOTHER DAY, ANOTHER CHILDBIRTH

—ALY—

Eleven days after Vera was born, Karen called to let us know she was heading to the hospital. I could tell from her voice that she was in a lot of pain. I remember thinking, *I've been there, sister!* Our parents stayed with Genevieve and Vera while Josh and I grabbed our "Lydia bag"—the separate hospital bag we'd packed and set aside for *this* birth—and rushed out to go get the last Taylor baby.

When we got to the hospital, we learned Karen's epidural had been delayed—but she was beyond ready for it. Apparently everyone and their momma (pun intended) decided to converge on that hospital's labor and delivery ward that morning, and there were no rooms left. They were holding Karen in triage until they could get her into a delivery room, and that triage area was burning up. As a fellow preggo just eleven days earlier, I knew the heat struggle is *real*! She was in a lot of pain and extremely uncomfortable until they were able to perform the epidural.

After that, Karen's whole demeanor changed and she was back to her happy, chatty self. The connection between us was so much greater now. Not only did I know her better, but I could now sympathize with what she was going through. Thinking back to my own pregnancy and birth experience, I couldn't imagine going through all that and then handing Vera over to another couple to raise. But that's exactly what Karen was doing. She knew it was the right thing for the baby, and she was making the courageous decision—again—to set her own feelings aside and focus on the child. I was in awe of her strength.

We thought we'd have a little time after the epidural, especially since Karen wasn't even in a regular room yet. However, when the doctor checked her again, he said she was ready to push. I thought, *We've been at the hospital less than an hour and it's already time to push?* We would have missed this if we hadn't moved to Kentucky for the month; there was no way we would have gotten there on time, especially since Karen went into labor almost a week before her due date.

Karen pushed a few times with our encouragement and tears, and then we saw Lydia Joyce Taylor enter the world. I sobbed and sobbed at God's faithfulness. It's not every day that a woman gets to watch her own daughter enter the world. We were overjoyed. Another perfect baby. Another miracle. Another answered prayer. We were all one big, happy family crowded around Lydia. It might have seemed awkward to onlookers, but Josh and I dearly loved this family who had given us two precious gifts. We all took turns taking pictures with Lydia, hugging, and crying together. At one point Karen leaned in to Josh and me and said some of the sweetest words I've ever heard: "Thank you. I am so thankful for you, and I'm honored to give Lydia to you."

That was such an incredible day. After all our plans, hopes, dreams, travel, relocation, health and job concerns, nosey television crews, and logistic nightmares, we were finally a family of five. Everything had gone off without a hitch (allergic reactions notwithstanding). Or so we thought.

CHAPTER 12

THY WILL BE DONE

—JOSH—

I was so blessed to be able to watch all three of my daughters come into the world. Each birth was life-changing and awe-inspiring—even though the second and third were just eleven days apart. Lydia's birth was just as miraculous as the other two, and everyone present could feel the love in the room. Sharing that moment with Karen and her family was incredible; everyone had time with the baby, and Aly and I took turns having skin-to-skin contact. I'm pretty sure we were covered in Vera's spit-up, so Lydia got a good dose of her sister too. Oh, newborn life!

As we mentioned, when Genevieve was born, Aly and I were able to get a hospital room a few doors down from Karen. That room had been a precious gift, especially in those first days when Karen started wavering in her decision to give up Genevieve for adoption. We hoped to have the same situation in Kentucky after Lydia's birth, but the hospital was too full. Karen finally got into a regular room after delivering Lydia in a triage room, but there weren't any beds available for Aly and me. We struggled with this; we couldn't fathom leaving the hospital without Lydia.

After sweating it out for what felt like forever, some of the nurses we had gotten to know figured out a solution: there was a room we could stay in; it just didn't have a bed. "Yes!" we said without a second thought. We just wanted to be close to Lydia. We didn't care what the conditions were. So we slept on the cold, tile hospital floor that night. The almost-empty room also had one hard waiting room chair and another one that somewhat reclined, so we rotated in and out of those too. Our Lydia was able to sleep in there with us for part of the night, so Aly held her in her arms while trying to sleep in an uncomfortable, unforgiving hospital chair. The conditions weren't ideal, but we didn't care. We were thankful to soak up every minute we could with the third Taylor baby girl.

—ALY—

What a night. I still had stomach cramping from Vera's birth, and that tile floor was *not* helping. However, when the nurse came in at 1:00 a.m. and asked if we wanted Lydia in our room, everything seemed perfect. I cuddled with her, sang to her, prayed for her, smelled her, and told her how much we adored her. It was the most uncomfortable, most wonderful night of my life. We were aching to get her home and join the rest of the family, but we still had to wait the two days before we could legally remove her from the hospital. Even after that, per Kentucky law, we had to wait three more days before the adoption became final. However, the birth family had already signed the papers to give us temporary custody until everything was finalized five days after the birth. That made the miserable hospital floor bearable. It was a small price to pay, and we knew we'd all be home just a couple of days later and Lydia would be with us forever.

We spent the entire next day with her. The nurses were so kind to us and did everything they could to make us comfortable and give us some privacy. They even partitioned off part of their nurses' station for us so we could soak in every sound, smile, and feeding. Josh and I kept marveling at how smoothly everything was going this time around. We were literally having a conversation about that when a social worker came in to talk with us. That was nothing unusual. Parents who adopt have to have a million conversations with doctors, lawyers, counselors, social workers, and everyone else under the sun during those crucial few days between the birth and the birth parents signing the final adoption papers. The social worker asked us how we were doing, and we said, "Great!" As any proud parent does, we took the opportunity to show off our little newborn girl. She then said she'd just left Karen's room, and we asked how she was doing.

"Not well," was the reply.

We were shocked—not that Karen was struggling some, but that she hadn't said anything to us. We'd seen her several times since the birth, and she was always smiling and laughing with us. Then the social worker dropped a bomb. She explained that Karen was trying to find a way to keep Lydia. We couldn't believe this was happening *again*. When this happened with Genevieve, I was genuinely surprised. As much as we had been warned about the possibility of adoption failure, I couldn't fathom it. This time, though, it felt like a sick joke. We had been with Karen off and on all day, and she hadn't even hinted that she was wavering on her decision. It was so frustrating! I could understand her having second thoughts; what I couldn't understand was why she hadn't been honest with us about it, especially after everything we'd already been through together. I assumed she was just scared to tell us.

We asked if we could talk to Karen ourselves, and she said we could. So, with tears filling our eyes, Josh and I started the long walk down the hall. As we went, we prayed for Lydia's future and for wisdom in how to handle whatever we were walking into. We went into Karen's room with Lydia in my arms and found her weeping. She confirmed what the social worker told us, apologizing over and over but being clear that she wanted to keep Lydia and was trying to figure out how she could do it. I was overwhelmed with so many emotions all at once. I was angry, but my heart also broke for this young woman who was obviously having a hard time.

Mainly, though, I wanted to remind her of all the reasons she had chosen adoption in the first place.

We sat in that hospital room for hours, talking through every detail and trying to figure out what was best for the baby. I couldn't bear the thought of losing Lydia. I knew in my spirit that I was her mommy from the moment I heard about her almost nine months earlier.

At the end of that conversation in her hospital room, there was no doubt or ambiguity: Karen was going to try and keep Lydia, and we were no longer going to adopt her. All the while, this perfect baby was still sleeping in my arms. Getting up after that talk and laying Lydia in the hospital bed was the hardest thing I have ever done in my life. I didn't want to let her go. Lydia's birth family were all staring at us, and we were staring at her. We stood there crying our eyes out, not knowing what to do or say. We loved her so much. This was *our daughter*, but we were supposed to leave her in that room and walk away forever? How was that possible? Josh asked if everyone would step out for a moment so we could have a few more minutes alone with our Lydia. After everything Josh and I had been through, this was the worst moment of our lives.

—JOSH—

I can't think back to those last few moments with Lydia without falling to my knees and getting sick to my stomach. It breaks my heart every single time it pops into my mind. Moments before, we were laughing and telling her all about her sisters. Then we were told she wasn't ours and that we had to leave her in the hospital. Indescribable. I have never sobbed that loudly or that long in my life. I was completely broken. I didn't know how I'd have the strength to physically walk away from my child.

Aly and I stood over her bed and prayed for Lydia. We felt as though we were handing her over to an unknown future, but I remember God speaking to me and assuring me that He still had her in His hands. Even though she wouldn't be with us, she would still be with Him. Eventually Aly and I knew it was time to go. We had to forcibly pull each other out of that room. We held hands and cried over this precious baby, told her how much we adored her and how we would keep doing our part to fight for her, and then we surrendered her to the Lord's care and protection. That moment—that *horrific* moment—is forever etched in my mind.

—ALY—

Standing there, praying over Lydia, I knew I had to let her go and entrust her to the Lord. It was torture, but I heard God clearly say to me, "Aly, you aren't her Savior. I am." I was blown away by that thought. It's hard for a mother to hear, but it is true. God could bless Lydia through anyone. Yes, I thought we were chosen to be hers and she was chosen to be ours, but maybe I'd been wrong the whole time.

Josh and I pulled each other away and gathered our things. The temporary custody order was revoked, and at this point there was no reason for us to be at the hospital and no reason for the nurses to accommodate us. In a flash we had gone from being Lydia's parents to being . . . well . . . *nothing*. We left in a daze, and neither of us had the strength to call our family to tell them what had happened. Back at our rental house, we had a houseful of grandparents and babies—all waiting to meet the newest addition to the Taylor family. We just weren't ready to bring them the same pain we were feeling at that moment. Besides, neither of us was in any shape to answer the endless questions we knew they'd ask. Instead, we drove around for a while and eventually ended up at the mall. We went in and walked around just like we'd done a couple of weeks earlier when we were trying to convince Vera to come out and meet the family. Only this time we weren't trying to coax a baby out; we were trying to understand how we would live *without* a baby.

I walked around that mall like a zombie. I was numb, then mad, then sad, then sick, then numb again. The cycle went on and on, and I'm sure my postpartum hormones weren't helping anything. I mindlessly wandered into a shoe store, and a happy, friendly, unsuspecting employee walked up to me and said, "How are you doing today, ma'am?" I'm typically pretty good at putting a smile on my face when I need to, even when I don't feel like it. But not today. Not now. The filter was gone, and I didn't care what I said or who I said it to.

"Horribly. I'm doing horribly."

The shoe salesman didn't know what to do. He muttered an apology and excused himself. My heart was empty. I missed my girls. I knew I'd see Genevieve and Vera within an hour or two. But Lydia . . . I didn't think I'd ever see my Lydia again. How could I live the rest of my life with this hole in my heart, this missing piece reserved only for that wonderfully unique little girl we had to leave in a Kentucky hospital? I couldn't wrap my mind around it, and I wasn't even beginning to accept it.

—JOSH—

I was shocked when Aly snapped at the salesman. I've known her since she was fourteen, and I'd never seen her be rude to anybody—intentionally or otherwise. I was worried about her and could tell she was almost at her breaking point. I wanted so badly to protect her from all this, but there was nothing I could do. After an hour of walking around the mall, we knew it was time to head home. We had to tell our family the tragic news. We were coming home empty-handed, without Lydia.

TRYING TO CARRY ON

We texted the family before we got home to give them a heads-up so they knew what to expect. When we got there we unpacked the whole story. As we told it we realized there weren't many details to share. Lydia was ours. Now she wasn't. That was pretty much it. We had uprooted our family, left

Aly's normal doctor, delivered Vera out of state, brought our families up to join us for a while, and now it was time for all of us to go back home, without Lydia. It was all so mind-boggling and soul-crushing.

I want to add here that we love Karen and her family. That has never changed, and it never will. We were devastated, but I don't want to discount their devastation either. I can't imagine how it would feel to carry a baby for nine months and then entrust her to someone else. We know it killed her to have to break our hearts. We know it was unexpected for her, and she never would have done anything to intentionally hurt us. She was just trying to figure out what the best thing was for her and Lydia. Birth parents are heroes to me. They are some of the most incredible, courageous people on the planet, and I will never say a bad word about the woman who had given us Genevieve. In fact, as we talked to our whole family, none of us ever got mad at her; instead, we were all just incredibly broken.

After we shared all the details, there was nothing left to say. We sat there quietly for a while, not sure what we were supposed to do next.

Before bed that night, Aly and I discussed the parable of the lost sheep in Luke 15:1–7. In that story, Jesus talked about a shepherd watching one hundred sheep who realized one was is missing. The good shepherd, Jesus said, left the ninety-nine to pursue the one who was lost. We felt like Lydia was our lost sheep. Yes, we had a wonderful family and we had been blessed with two amazing baby girls. But there was one missing. That thought occupied my mind throughout that entire sleepless night. I felt like God was telling me to fight for the missing sheep until the very end.

In that situation, the "very end" would be the fifth day after Lydia's birth, the day when Karen was originally supposed to sign the final adoption papers. I discussed it with Aly the next morning, and we decided we'd stay in Kentucky and fight for our lost sheep, even if *fighting* simply meant waiting. Lord knows we had done our share of waiting and praying over the past few years; this was a battle we knew how to fight. So we told the family we wanted to stay in Kentucky until Lydia was discharged from the hospital and the adoption deadline had passed. We wanted to demonstrate our faithfulness to the Lord by doing everything He called us to do in adopting this little girl. He had called us to stay until that fifth day, and that's what we were going to do. And if we still went home without Lydia after that, at least we would always know we fought until the end.

—ALY—

Those final days in Kentucky were hard. We tried going to back to the hospital a few more times, but we didn't have a right to visit Lydia. That's hard to even type more than two years later. *How do I not have the right to see my baby?* I thought. I couldn't stop thinking of Lydia as mine. The law, however, saw things differently. Legally, we had no connection. But in my heart we were forever bound to each other.

We went to church the Sunday after she was born. We had been blessed with a great congregation during our short time in Kentucky, and the pastor and his wife knew that we were there to adopt a baby. After church, the pastor came up and congratulated us, asking about Lydia. We broke down crying. It hit us that we had texted him when she was born, but we hadn't followed up when the adoption fell apart. I wanted to live in denial, to be able to say Lydia was great and was waiting for us to pick her up from the hospital. But I had to tell the truth. Through tears, I explained that we didn't have Lydia, we *weren't getting* Lydia, and we were planning on heading home Tuesday without her. No matter how many times I explained the situation to someone, it still didn't feel real.

We struggled through the rest of Sunday and then Monday. Monday was surrender day for me. That Monday night I completely surrendered Lydia to the Lord. I had been holding on so tight all week to the idea that she was ours. I still hadn't been able to imagine our life without her or her life without us. But as I prayed that last night in Kentucky, I felt something release in my spirit. I realized I wasn't releasing Lydia; I was releasing *control*. I knew the issue was out of my hands. There was nothing I could do except trust that God would care for Lydia no matter where she was or who she was with.

Finally, Tuesday arrived. That day was the bookend to what had started out as a wonderful new chapter for our lives but was now ending so terribly. We struggled with how we would possibly go home and move on with our lives. The social worker called and told us the birth family would allow us to come to the hospital and see Lydia one last time before she was discharged. We were so grateful for that act of kindness. Again, we loved this family; we were just heartbroken over the situation.

THY WILL BE DONE

—JOSH—

An ironic side note, the Hillary Scott song "Thy Will" was popular on Christian radio at this time, and it seemed like we heard that song a hundred times a day during our last week in Kentucky. It came on the radio all the time, and my mom basically kept it playing on a loop on her phone. I guess that's what we were all praying for Lydia that week, for God's will to be done. Too often I think people use that prayer to make them feel better about giving up or losing. Or they say, "Thy will be done" as part of their acceptance process when something doesn't go the way they wanted it to go.

I've done both of those plenty of times, but this time was different. I didn't pray for God's will to be done as a way of giving up; I prayed it as I fought for it. I believe praying for God's will has as much to do with *fighting* for His will as it does with *accepting* the results when all is said and done. That's why we stayed in Kentucky until that Tuesday. Tuesday was the last day adoption protocol laws would be in effect. That's why we kept going back to the hospital to check on Lydia. That's why we stayed in touch with the birth family. That's why we were in constant contact with the attorneys and social workers. We did everything we could to show everyone involved how much we loved that little girl. Even though we were told the adoption was over, we made it clear that we were still in Kentucky and we were ready to get her at any point.

When we woke up that morning knowing we were going to be able to see Lydia one last time, we were grateful for all God had done and continued to do in our lives. We cherished the two daughters we were taking home, and we wouldn't trade those few days we had spent with Lydia for anything. We wanted her so badly, but God had finally started to bring us a sense of peace that He would provide for her in a mighty way.

—ALY—

When we arrived at the hospital, we were led to the same room that had become our makeshift hospital room the day after Lydia was born. We had been there such a short time, but it held so many memories for us. And now this was apparently where we'd say our last goodbye to Lydia.

After a few minutes, the door opened and a nurse wheeled that precious baby back into "our" room. This time, however, I was choosing joy, doing my best to soak up every moment we had with Lydia. The nurses were so kind and gracious to us during this visit. Their smiles, glances, handholds, and prayers meant the world to us on a very difficult day. I could tell they loved Lydia too. They kept going on and on about what a great baby she was and how she never cried. They also told me she hadn't been drinking her bottle well since we left, so they asked if I could feed her. Of course! The nurses were amazed that she sucked it right down without a fuss; she apparently hadn't done that the whole time. Cue the tears! I was trying so hard not to lose it. I had to keep reminding myself that she wasn't ours. *But she is!* my mind kept screaming.

Josh and I took turns holding her, feeding her, changing her diaper, and doing all the other things parents do with their newborn. We had been in there with her for more than an hour, and we kept expecting someone to walk in and tell us it was time to go. We were prepared for that, but we certainly weren't going to initiate leaving. It was fine if they needed to kick us out, but they'd have to tell us to do it!

Eventually the door cracked open and a woman we hadn't seen before stepped in. She was well-dressed and had an air of authority about her, so we assumed she was there to ask us to leave. Instead, she said, "I need y'all to hold tight. There have been a few changes that are happening at your attorney's office. I just need you to hold tight a bit."

What? What is happening? What in the world does "hold tight" mean? My mind was racing. Josh and I were scrambling to figure out what was happening, but it didn't make sense. Of course, we hoped and prayed that this somehow meant we'd be able to take Lydia home with us, but we couldn't imagine how so many things could have changed in the past hour. We honestly couldn't take any more disappointments, so we desperately tried not to get our hopes up too high, but we couldn't help it. I may have looked calm on the outside, but on the inside, I was screaming!

—JOSH—

That was one of the craziest moments of my life. It was as if the woman who came in to talk to us was speaking in code or something, like she had just received a critical piece of information that she couldn't share quite yet. I enjoy intrigue as much as the next guy, but this was not the time for mysteries! Too much was on the line, and Aly and I just about lost our minds waiting in that little hospital room.

I tried to talk myself down. I told myself it was probably another form that needed to be signed or another conversation we had to have with the social worker as a type of postmortem on the failed adoption, or maybe the birth family wanted to see us one last time to say goodbye. I had no clue.

Aly and I probably thought of a hundred different scenarios, but we were only praying for one. *Lord, if it is Your will, please let her be ours.*

—ALY—

Josh and I literally said nothing the entire time. We just sat there with our mouths open and minds swimming. We kept looking at each other and squeezing each other's hands as if to say, *I'm freaking out! What do you think is happening?* Finally, as I tried (and failed) to silence the dance party that had broken out in my head, my phone buzzed in my purse. I held Lydia with one arm and reached into my purse with the other. Pulling my phone up to my face, I saw that it was a text from Karen. We hadn't heard from her since we'd left the hospital a few days earlier except for one short thank-you text she sent in reply to one of my messages checking on her. The text I was looking at now, though, wasn't a simple "thank you." It was long. And miraculous.

Karen explained that she had thought long and hard over the past several days about what was best for Lydia. As much as she wanted to keep Lydia, she had come to realize that Josh and I were the best thing for her. She told us how difficult the decision was, but she also knew it was the right thing. She was certain. In fact, she was texting us from the attorney's office—and she said she was in the process of signing the adoption papers.

Just like that, Lydia was ours.

Josh and I burst into tears. Another couple in the nursery room with us offered to take a picture, capturing the moment we learned Lydia would be our daughter forever. I was a wreck, praising God and thinking over and over, *Did this really just happen?* There are no words for what I felt in that moment. What we knew and sensed from the beginning had come to pass. Lydia was worth the fight, the tears, the confusion, the surrender, the hard tile floor, the devastating discussions. She was worth it. Our lost little sheep was coming home.

They asked us to bring the car seat upstairs so they could strap her in, but we didn't have her car seat with us. It was still in our Kentucky home where we'd left it that morning. When we came to the hospital, we never dreamed we'd actually be able to bring her home with us. Genevieve's car seat was in the car, though, so Josh ran down to check it. Fortunately, it was rated for babies down to five pounds, and Lydia was five pounds and four ounces. Perfect! We also didn't have any clothes for her. Again, why would we? Lydia was dressed in a little white hospital shirt and a tiny white hospital hat with a crooked bow on it. I so badly wanted to put her in one of the cute newborn outfits we had, but we had nothing. No outfit, no hat, no newborn car seat—but we had *her*. We figured we would be walking out of the hospital empty-handed; instead, I was triumphantly escorted out in a wheelchair holding Lydia just as I had been two weeks earlier with Vera. I was a mommy—again!

—JOSH—

God did it again.

I don't know why He has continued to work in our lives in such big ways, but we are so incredibly thankful He has. I also find it no coincidence that we had finally surrendered the situation fully into God's hand just the night before. We knew He would take care of Lydia, and we were beyond thrilled to now know for sure that *we* were part of His plan for her. The beauty and miracle of adoption will never cease to amaze me!

THE MAGIC OF TELEVISION

It's weird to think that television crews were still hanging around for all this drama. Once we knew the adoption *wasn't* happening, the network pulled most of the cameramen and producers, mostly for privacy's sake. Fortunately, they decided to leave a few people with us in Kentucky to capture our final few days there and to interview us about having to say goodbye to Lydia. They weren't with us at the hospital, but we knew they were at the house to film us returning home without the baby we'd hoped to adopt.

When we left the hospital, Aly and I made one of the best decisions of our lives: we called the camera crew to tell them what happened. Stunned by the turn of events and knowing they had TV gold, they made one request: "Can you keep it from your parents until you get home? We'd love to get their genuine surprise when you walk in with the baby." Of course we said yes. Our family had walked with us through so much heartache over the years and especially this past week; the idea of giving them one shocking moment of pure joy was thrilling. We knew we would catch them completely off guard. The car seat and all Lydia's clothes were still with them at the house, and we had been given every indication that it was all over.

The camera crew had our parents sitting at the kitchen table with Genevieve and Vera when we drove up. They wanted to make sure no one saw us get Lydia out of the car. The crew told our family that we would be coming in to talk to them about how our "final" visit with Lydia went and how it felt to say goodbye. When everything was ready, Aly and I made our way to the kitchen with Lydia in our arms. Our hearts were pounding a million beats a minute as we walked around the corner and said, "Surprise!"

Our parents lost it. My dad was the first to see us and let out a big, "Oh my gracious!" Aly's mom jumped up from her seat and stood there covering her face in shock. My mom was holding Vera and she stood up shaking. No one could believe it. They all rushed over to check out the beautiful baby in Aly's arms. Genevieve, who had been over the moon for Vera over the past two weeks, was able to meet her *new* little sister. Everyone was chattering and praising God, and Aly just kept saying, "I know! I know! I know!" Then I got to see the most important women in my life—my incredible wife, her mother, my mom, and my three beautiful little girls—all together for the first time. It was one of the most amazing moments of our lives, and I can relive it on video any time I want!

As crazy as life under the reality TV microscope had been at times, this moment made it all worth it.

CHAPTER 13

CELEBRATE THE MIRACLES

—ALY—

I can't believe this is my life! When we got home with Vera and Lydia, I had to pinch myself. To go from not knowing if I would live, to being declared cancer-free, then to being home with my three miracle girls is just too much to take at times. When people hear our story, they are always blown away by what God has done in our family. I don't blame them. I've lived this whole adventure, and I'm still blown away by it! However, it's important to remember that our story isn't perfect and it isn't over yet. It's easy for people to hear everything we've been through and assume that all our problems are over, that we've conquered every obstacle and fought every battle. We haven't. The Taylor Five has had quite an adventure, but we're not fading away into the happily ever after quite yet.

We still have to deal with issues from having gone through cancer, infertility, and adoption. We never let our struggles overpower our blessings, but we want to be real with others about not only the battles we've won but also the ones we're still fighting. That kind of honesty and vulnerability is so important, even for a private person like me. We have so many tools and opportunities these days for living authentic lives in public, but too often we hide behind our highlight reels. We use social media to show the very best parts of our lives and try to hide the mess. Social media rarely shows the difficult, ugly moments of life. But that's *real life* for all of us.

Reality TV has an especially bad reputation for painting fake pictures of people's lives. Some shows make people look really, really good, and other shows make people look really, really bad. That's one of the things that made me so nervous about going on *Rattled*. I didn't want to show the world an unrealistic view of our lives; I wanted to show people the real thing. Fortunately, TLC felt the same way. Josh and I originally thought the show would just film us in Kentucky and stop when we brought the girls home. However, they were interested in seeing our *whole* life, warts and all.

After they filmed us a couple of times once we got Vera and Lydia home, the producers asked what else we had coming up in our *regular* life. We mentioned that we were coming up on the five-year mark of my cancer diagnosis and explained how significant that was. My chance of a recurrence dropped dramatically at the two-year mark, and those chances would fall down to the basement at year five. They asked if they could hang out with us a while longer and film that doctor visit. We were honestly surprised that TLC was so interested in this, but I immediately said, "Oh my, yes! Of course!" I loved the idea of having this appointment on video. I knew it would be something my kids could look back on for years to come. I was also excited about putting an encouraging message of hope on national television for viewers who were struggling through their own cancer battles. That was one of the reasons Josh and I had agreed to do the show in the first place, so there was no way I was going to pass up an opportunity to document my five-year cancer-free celebration for all to see.

GRADUATING FROM CANCER

When I was first diagnosed, I talked to several cancer patients. I needed wisdom and insight, and I needed some idea of what I was up against. One of the first people I talked to was a breast cancer survivor who was a few years past her diagnosis. She stressed over and over how much she couldn't wait to hit the five-year mark. She said she felt like she was holding her breath until she got there. Soon after, I talked to a woman who was only a few months into her cancer journey. She told me she was already planning the huge celebration she would have after her five-year milestone. Then I talked to another survivor who was fifteen years past her diagnosis, and she said one of the happiest days of her life was the day she hit the five-year mark. You can see the theme here, right? In the cancer world, few days are more significant than the fifth anniversary from your diagnosis. Even in those first days of my journey, before I even knew what type and stage of cancer I had, I started focusing on that five-year mark. I knew it would be a big deal and something I would *definitely* celebrate.

When I first got to MD Anderson and learned how serious my cancer was and how it had already spread to my lymph nodes, I tried to keep my eyes on that five-year goal. We avoided statistics as much as possible, but that was one marker we held on to. *If I can make it to five years*, I realized, *I'll trust I have beaten this thing for good.* Then came the chemo, surgery, radiation, and reconstruction nightmare.

I was diagnosed on October 17, 2011. Once I realized how important the five-year mark was, I joked that I wished there was a five-year sleeping pill. Little did I know how many wonderful things would happen in my life in those five years! But if I could have been knocked out cold at the start of my journey and woken up on October 17, 2016, I probably would have done it. It was hard to imagine back then what the next five years would look like. It was all so scary, like I was stepping into a dark cloud. I knew I was starting a long race, and the five-year mark was the finish line. I just didn't know how I'd have the strength to make it there.

Now, on the other side of the journey looking back, I know there's only one way I made it: Jesus. Josh was an incredible partner, and my family was amazing. However, I would not have gotten through it without my Comforter and Healer, Jesus Christ.

My five-year appointment was originally scheduled for Halloween, but my doctor had to reschedule. Can you guess what day they moved the appointment to? October 17. That's the day my life changed forever in 2011, and that was going to be the day I'd know for sure that the cancer was *gone* in 2016. I felt like God had given me a gift when they changed my appointment. I had a great sense that He wanted to frame this whole thing in the little five-year box I'd imagined in my head. Thank God I didn't sleep through the previous five years. He saw me through to the end, and it was time to get the official word on my cancer status.

Josh and I left the girls with our parents and friends, and we set off for Houston the same way we started this journey—just the two of us. It was a great opportunity for us to spend some quality (and quiet) time together without three babies demanding our attention. We spent a lot of time thinking, talking, and praying about all that had happened over the previous five years. We slept a lot (no kids!), and we cried a lot. I trusted that I was healed, but I still had a flood of anxiety pour over me in Houston. There were so many memories there. So many bad doctor reports, test results, surgeries, and treatments. It felt overwhelming to be back there having tests run and waiting for my oncologist to deliver what I knew would be life-changing news—one way or another.

When my oncologist came into the exam room, she was almost in tears as she went over the significance of this appointment. I love her so much; she and I had walked such a long journey together, and I couldn't have asked for a better guide. She examined me, asked a ton of questions, wrote a lot of notes, and ran a few tests. Finally, with the biggest smile on her face, she said, "Aly, I'm happy to tell you that you have graduated to the survivorship section of the hospital!" Survivorship! She went on to explain that she no longer needed to see me. It was weird to think of not seeing her again, but there was no *reason* for her to see me. She sees *cancer patients*, and, praise God, that wasn't me anymore. And it will never be me again, in Jesus's name.

TIME TO CELEBRATE

I had graduated from college three times by that point, first with my bachelor's, then my master's, then my PhD. But none of those can hold a candle to the fourth graduation of my adult life—graduating from cancer. I wasn't sure what to do. I'd dreamt of this day for so long, and here it was. The only thing I knew to do was celebrate. We had a big party when I hit the two-year mark, and we all agreed we'd have an even bigger one when I got to five years. Well, here we were!

It was impossible not to think back to our little celebration on Josh's twenty-seventh birthday when we first got to Houston five years earlier. I remembered my shock and joy when my mom and I walked up and saw confetti all over our table. We took that as a miracle back then, as God giving us a clear reminder that He was there with us during those dark days.

Now I truly believe that was a prophetic moment where God told me there would be many celebrations to come. I also believe it was His way of reminding me to celebrate every moment. I remember thinking, praying, and hoping that there would be lots of celebrating in my future—even though it felt like we had no reason to celebrate then. Well, we had reason to celebrate *now*. Josh and I had made it through the dark cloud. Our faith was stronger, our relationship was closer, our family was bigger, and I had beaten cancer. Time to party!

—JOSH—

That five-year "cancerversary" party was surreal. It was the perfect bookend to the prayer-filled send-off gathering our friends had for us the night before we left for our first appointment in Houston. Almost everyone from that send-off came back to celebrate Aly's five-year mark with us. Looking across the crowd of people and remembering how important each of them had been along the way was priceless. Our friends Amy and Ron had sung songs of praise at the send-off five years earlier, and now they were singing songs of praise to honor what God had done in our lives. Everything had come full circle.

We were also glad that TLC asked to film the party. This is another blessing, to have these key moments captured professionally on film. This footage will be a treasure for our family for the rest of our lives. TLC used the party in the season finale of *Rattled*, ending the season by celebrating all four of my miracle girls. A few years before, when we had Aly's two-year party, a friend commented that she was praying we'd have a little Taylor baby running around by the time we had the five-year party. Who could have imagined that, three years later, we'd have not one but *three* perfect Taylor babies?

—ALY—

There's one thing for certain about the Taylor family: we will celebrate like no other. God has given us so many reasons to celebrate, and we want to be faithful in remembering both the good and bad. We honor the valleys He has walked us through, and we rejoice in the victories. I don't care who you are or what is going on in your life; you can find *some* reason to celebrate.

Like I said earlier, this doesn't mean our story is over. The five-year celebration capped off one major phase of our life, but we still have plenty of living left to do. And, to be honest, we're still healing from what happened during those five years. They were hard, hard times. Years have passed, but the wounds are still fresh. There are days when I think I'm good, but something will happen that sends me back in time to a deeply emotional, painful place. I'll get a new pain in my body and a flash of fear will come over me that the cancer has returned. I'll get a whiff of "chemo smell" (you know what I mean if you've been through it), and I'll get physically ill. Someone will make a flippant statement about cancer or death, and I'll feel myself get angry. I'll hear of a friend's or acquaintance's new cancer diagnosis, and my heart will break for that person. Yes, I'm *healed* . . . but that healing doesn't mean I'm not also still broken. I'm both.

Josh reminds me that it's all part of the continual cycle of brokenness and healing. I have full faith that God has healed me, but I also know I need to walk in that healing every day. There are days when I *feel* broken and plenty of days when I *am* broken. But God is always there to put those broken pieces back together again, continually remaking me into something new. In those times I can hear Him whisper, "You are healed, My child. But you are still healing. Depend on Me. Hide My Word in your heart. Speak it out loud. Abide in Me. I offer healing—over and over and over again."

—JOSH—

We are all so incredibly blessed, but we must not get lost in our bliss and think we don't need God anymore. Instead, we must continually live lives of desperation—desperate *for* Him and dependent *on* Him each and every day. We were desperate for God during our cancer battle. We were desperate for God during our infertility and adoption struggles. And now, as the parents of three little girls, we are desperate for Him in an entirely different way. We are desperate for Him to empower us to raise three warriors for His kingdom. If that doesn't bring you to your knees in desperation, praying for guidance on how to raise little souls, I don't know what will.

Our prayer is that we always remember what God has done for us, that we continually celebrate His goodness, that we are honest with our shortcomings and struggles, and that we give our testimony as often as we can. Our pain has not been in vain, and we strive to give other people the hope that we have experienced in Christ Jesus. Psalm 78:1-8 declares:

In you, LORD, I have taken refuge;
 let me never be put to shame.
In your righteousness, rescue me and deliver me;
 turn your ear to me and save me.
Be my rock of refuge,
 to which I can always go;
give the command to save me,
 for you are my rock and my fortress.
Deliver me, my God, from the hand of the wicked,
 from the grasp of those who are evil and cruel.

For you have been my hope, Sovereign LORD,
 my confidence since my youth.
From birth I have relied on you;
 you brought me forth from my mother's womb.
 I will ever praise you.
I have become a sign to many;
 you are my strong refuge.
My mouth is filled with your praise,
 declaring your splendor all day long.

God has truly been our rock since the beginning, and our mouths will *always* be filled with His praise, declaring His splendor all day long.

CHAPTER 14

EMBRACING DESTROYED PLANS

—JOSH—

I have to laugh whenever I think back to the life we imagined before cancer. It's shocking how naïve we were back then about who we were, what we wanted, and what we thought really mattered. If all the things I'd hoped for and dreamed of when we first got married had come true, I probably would have been happy and fulfilled. But I'd have no idea how much joy I'd be missing out on. God absolutely shattered our plans. He broke them into a million tiny pieces. And I am in awe of the incredible life He gave us instead. The life we have today is better than anything we ever could have hoped for ourselves, and God did it by breaking us.

—ALY—

I thought I had everything figured out back then. My life plan made sense. It was a clear, simple, straight line from where we were to where we thought we wanted to go. What we didn't realize, however, is that God rarely draws a straight line when He's mapping out our lives. There are all these twists and turns we never expect and, honestly, never want to take. Only He knows where it all leads, though. He used every heartache, every health scare, every surgery, every treatment, every bad doctor's report, and every fertility frustration to weave a beautiful tapestry—one I never could have envisioned when I was twenty-four. Yes, I'm a planner. I map out my days, and I love making lists. But God has taught me not to be so rigid about my plans anymore. If His plans are truly better than our own (and they are), then I want mine destroyed.

EMBRACE YOUR STORY

These days I try to think of life in terms of a story rather than a plan. That hasn't always been the case, though. After Josh's moment with God where he surrendered control over what happens to our lives, Josh's outlook turned 180 degrees. He was equally, if not at times more optimistic than I was! I remember many times throughout our journey when something terrible would happen—like another failed month trying to get pregnant or a weird side effect from my cancer treatment—and Josh would say something like, "Maybe this is just part of our story." Gag! It was often infuriating to hear him meet so many challenges with this optimism. The worst one, I think, was when we were expecting the call from the fertility doctor to tell us if our IVF had worked. Remember, we set up a video camera to record the good news, but instead we were left with a video of one of the darkest days of our lives. After crying with Josh on the sofa for a while, I looked up and noticed the camera. I said, "Oh, Josh! Did you know this was still recording?"

He looked at me and said, "Yes. I knew whatever we heard, good or bad, would be part of our story." Gag again!

Today, after seeing how God has arranged all these pieces into such an incredible life, I have to admit Josh was right: all those things *were* part of our story. And as I move forward as a woman, wife, and mother, I want to fully embrace the story God is telling about our family. I encourage you to do the same. Whoever you are, wherever you are, and whatever is going on in your life right now, you are *unique*. God is crafting a personal, powerful, wonderfully original story just for you.

We all live so much of our lives trying *not* to embrace our story. You might say, "Aly, if you only knew my story, you'd be telling me to run from it, not embrace it!" You're probably right. That's why I never say it to someone in their moment of pain. I know from experience it may do more harm than good. Trust me, I *never* wanted to hear it from Josh when I was balled up on the couch in tears about some diagnosis or bad report. In fact, a few years ago, after I had passed my two-year cancer mark and as we were struggling through infertility, I wrote a blog post titled "This Is Just Part of Our Story"—one of Josh's favorite expressions. I took a few loving jabs at Josh in that post, but God was also giving me some perspective on what Josh was saying. Here's an excerpt:

November 9, 2014
I get tired of [all this] being a "part of our story." Why can't "our story" be one that is *typical*—free of sickness, hardship, trouble, infertility, pain, and worry? . . . I, of course, don't know the answer to why we have gone through suffering like we have. And yes, I wish our life was "easier." But I will embrace my story. If I just looked at my life and the hardships we've endured without trusting in my Creator and friend, I would literally crumble. Seriously.

I've known incredible pain and I've known immense joy. It is all part of my story. Because the pain has been so deep, I know the joy will be that much more.

Life is such a crazy ride. Glad I know *Who* is directing it, and yes, it's all a part of our story, even when I want to kick Josh for saying that.

I honestly don't know how God gave me the clarity to write, "Because the pain has been so deep, I know the joy will be that much more." Reading that years later, after I've seen Him bring these three beautiful girls into my life and get me safely past the five-year cancer-free celebration, I'm blown away by how true those words are. If it took going through that pain to get where I am today, I'd do every part of it again. If you're going through a season of darkness and loneliness right now, please trust that there is joy on the other side. Keep pressing on and know you're not alone! The Storyteller is doing something wonderful in your life, even if you can't read the whole story yet.

One warning, though: when I say, "Embrace your story," I want you to hear, "Embrace *your* story." In our social media–filled world, it's easy to fall into the trap of comparing your life to someone else's. I'm not just talking about wanting the *good* things someone else has. That's the standard social media/jealousy/discontentment trap we hear so much about. No, I'm talking about the opposite. When you're sick or struggling, it's easy to let someone else's *bad* news throw your own recovery into a tailspin.

When I was going through cancer, it was so tempting for me to compare my journey to someone else's—especially if that person had a similar diagnosis. I'd read about her situation and treatment plan and think, *She did [fill in the blank]. Maybe I should do that too.* While getting information from others was good, I had to constantly remind myself to stay focused on *my* journey.

I mentioned previously that the two breast cancer survivors who helped me through my treatments both had recurrences and ultimately passed away. Even now, another dear friend is battling breast cancer a second time. If I'm not careful, fear can overtake me. I can fall into thinking, *She's having a recurrence. She was clear at the five-year mark, but now she has it again. It could happen to me too.* No. I love my friend and I'm there to support her, but I'm not living *her* story; I'm living *mine.* I can't let her new fight steal the joy from my own healing.

The same was true for infertility. I would talk to someone who had tried a certain herb, medication, acupuncture, or fertility doctor and wonder if I should try it too. I spent countless hours on a site called BabyCenter, where I heard women around the world talk about ovulation, pregnancy, miscarriage, and birth stories. I realized I was constantly comparing myself to them and ultimately had to stop visiting the site for good because I had become obsessed with it.

It happened again during our adoption journey. We heard so many amazing stories, but people were also quick to fill our minds with their horror stories of failed adoptions. It was easy for us to live in fear, worried that what happened to them would happen to us. Again, we had to filter out those negative voices. We chose to focus on *our* story and trust that God would lead us where He wanted us. We were determined not to allow others' experiences to define our own.

My heart breaks for the trials others are going through, but Josh and I continually remind ourselves that we are living a different story—*our* story. We believe that I am completely healed and well, even though others have faced a recurrence. We believe that God completely protected my womb and gave us a miracle baby, even though others with the same infertility diagnosis never got pregnant. We believe our girls will be secure, loved, confident, and full of joy, even if others who adopted have had a different outcome. I'm not hiding my head in the sand and refusing to face reality; I'm doing the opposite—I'm living my reality and thanking God for it. I just won't let someone else's story derail my own, and neither should you.

CHOOSE JOY

Since we've been on *Rattled* for a couple of seasons now, people often recognize us and ask, "How are you guys so happy?" The show documented so many emotional—and often insane—moments in our life. Viewers have watched us cry a lot, but they also see us laugh and smile through it all.

So when people ask why we always seem so happy, I give them two answers. First, I tell them it's easy to be happy when we have so much to be thankful for. God has richly blessed our lives, and we will never fail to give Him glory for that. Second, I tell people that we simply *choose* joy. There was a time in our life when we felt anything *but* joyful, but here we are today, blessed beyond imagination. How could we *not* be joyful?

I want to be clear here, though. I'm not saying we're *always* happy. We definitely are not. My girls already know the difference between happiness and joy. I recently came home from a counseling conference and brought them some new fingernail polish. Genevieve got the biggest smile on her face and said, "Oh, Mom! I'm so happy!" Was she filled with joy over the nail polish? No, she simply felt a rush of happiness at my gift. Five minutes later, the thrill was gone, and she was back to normal.

Contrast that with our typical routine when I discipline her. When she disobeys, she often has to go into time-out for a little while. When her time's up, I walk over and ask her to apologize for whatever she did. But then, before she can get up, I ask, "Now, are you ready to choose joy?" Most of the time she lights up and says yes before running off. Other times she tells me she isn't ready to choose joy, and I tell her that once she is ready to choose it, she can get up. I use that wording intentionally, because I want them to know that joy is a choice, even in times of hardship or, in her case, in times of punishment. Joy isn't a *feeling*; it's an *outlook on life.* Of course I want my kids to be happy, but I don't pray for their happiness that much. Instead, I pray that they find their true, unending source of joy in Jesus Christ. They have to choose Him and choose to live in the joy He gives every day, no matter what the circumstances of their lives are at any given time.

Author and speaker John Bevere says, "The extent to which you suffer should be the extent to which you rejoice." This has been so true in our life. We have suffered much, and because of that, we rejoice much. Everyone wants the miracle moment, but you don't get the miracle without first facing the impossible. It's easy to choose joy when the miracle comes, but I challenge you to choose joy while you're still waiting. It won't always be easy or feel natural, but it's still your choice. Don't wait to *feel* it. *Choose* it.

PERSPECTIVE IS EVERYTHING

—JOSH—

Cancer gave us a perspective on life that we never would have had otherwise. I obviously wish we could have learned it some other way, but that's not the story God wanted to tell in, through, and for us. So we learned it through cancer. What we discovered through that journey is that people tend to worry and stress about so many things that ultimately don't matter. And when I say "people," I mean Josh Taylor. I can be a worrier. It is definitely something I have to constantly keep in check. Aly is the optimistic, glass-half-full one in our relationship. She can usually tell if something is *really* worth worrying about. Not me. I get so aggravated with myself when I worry about business and financial stuff, even after all the miracles I've watched God do. But—and this is important—I worry a heck of a lot less about that stuff than I used to. God's working on this part of me, constantly showing me that I can trust Him with whatever I'm worried about. If He can heal my wife's cancer, He can certainly fix a financial bump in the road.

When Aly became cancer-free, she and I made a pact that we would not get caught up in all the things the world gets caught up in. That may mean we never live in a nicer, bigger house. It may mean our kids aren't involved in a ton of activities. It may mean we'll always look weird to other people. Who cares? As Christians, aren't we *supposed* to stand out and look different from the world? We don't want to waste our time on things that don't matter; we'd rather pour our time and energy into things that honor God, advance His kingdom, and bring real joy into our lives. It's hard to do that if we're worrying about pesky little annoyances all the time.

Again, I'm still a work in progress on this, but fortunately, I have Aly keeping me on track. She told me recently that she doesn't even *believe* in bad days anymore. I love that perspective. Any day we're alive on this earth is a good day. Sure, bad things can happen (and often do), but every day we're here is one more day that God has blessed us with life and endless opportunities.

Our "Houston family," the Stanfills, made a huge impression on us during Aly's cancer treatments. We lived with them during much of our time in Houston, and we forged a bond that will last a lifetime. Before we left for the hospital each day, Tammy would always send us off with a hearty, "Make a great day!" I love the way she phrased it. She didn't say "Have a good day" or "I hope you have a good day." She was crystal clear: "*Make* a great day." She helped us understand that our perspective was our choice. We could choose to let the circumstances of life bring us down, or we could take her advice and make every day a great day. That's what we've tried to do every day since then, and that's what we're teaching our daughters to do.

SPEAK LIFE

—ALY—

Another huge lesson I learned during cancer was how powerful words can be. At church one Sunday during my treatments in Houston, I went down front for prayer. A kind lady partnered to pray with me, and I gave her a quick rundown on what I was going through. Then I asked for prayers for my complete healing. The woman looked me square in the eyes, grabbed my face with both hands, and said, "Darling, you *are* healed and you are whole." She was so certain; it was honestly a bit unsettling. I remember thinking, *Um, no, I'm not. I have cancer. Do you need to see the doctor's report?* But as she spoke, her message started to make sense to me. She continued,

"You must walk in faith, honey. You are healed. You are whole. I want you to start saying that. I want you to start saying that *out loud*. Will you do that?"

It took a huge step of faith, but I took her advice. I started telling myself—out loud—that I was healed. Over and over, every day I said, "Aly, you are healed. You are whole." Just saying my own words, spoken in faith, boosted my faith more than I can say. I started by *making* myself say it; then, over time, I actually started *believing* it. I discovered the truth of Proverbs 18:21: "The tongue has the power of life and death." That truth has changed my life.

At the risk of sounding overly dramatic, I believe you can change the course of your life with the power of your words. If you don't change anything about yourself except the words that come out of your mouth, your life would still be entirely different. Try it! It's not about false confidence or the power of positive thinking; it's about speaking words of life. I now do this with everything, especially my children.

I once feared that I talked about my kids too much, that I was simply bragging and being an obsessive mom. As I prayed about it, though, I realized I wasn't *bragging*; I was speaking words of life about them. I never want my children to doubt who they are. I want each of them to always remember what a miraculous treasure they are, so I tell them. A lot. I tell them what I see in them, and I tell them how God sees them. I brag to them and others about their character and God-given gifts. As they get older, I want those to be the things they hear from me. I'd rather fill their ears with *who they are*, not *what they can do*. Yes, we'll talk about grades and college. And if they can't carry a tune in a bucket, I'll probably suggest they not try out for *American Idol* or *The Voice*. But more than any of that, I will always tell them who they are in the eyes of their mom, their dad, and their heavenly Father.

—JOSH—

Because I'm naturally not as positive as Aly is, she'll correct me for saying something negative or for having a certain tone in my voice. Sometimes it's over-the-top, but I love that she's so concerned with the words we say and how we say them. She's helped me understand the weight of my words. I don't want to be the kind of person who always has a negative thing to say about others or certain situations. Instead, I want to speak in faith, saying words of life over my wife, kids, family, friends, work, and myself. My God is the God of the impossible, so why would I want my words to show otherwise? I want my words—*our words*—to change the world. I truly believe that they can.

THE BEST ADVICE I'VE EVER RECEIVED

—ALY—

I was writing in a journal about a year ago and came across this question: "What is the best advice you have ever received?" I really thought about this. I thought about my mom always telling me to "kill people with kindness." I thought about my high school Bible teacher teaching us about Jesus loving the least of these. I thought about our Houston mom, Tammy, always telling us to "Make a great day!" But then it hit me. I knew what the best piece of advice I ever received was. It came in one of my darkest moments and has brought me through every moment since.

When I was about a year out of my cancer treatment, I started having debilitating headaches. I wrote about this in an earlier chapter. One day I was lying in bed not wanting to move when my mother-in-law, Renea, called to check on me. I'm not sure if Josh told her to call me, or if she was calling to check on me on her own. When she asked how I was doing, I could tell she *really* wanted to know. So I asked her if we could go talk somewhere. Honestly, I was at the end of my rope, and I wanted some advice. I was in so much pain. I didn't know if I should go see another doctor, if I should try to pray it away, or if I was going crazy! I just needed someone to tell me what to do.

She picked me up and we drove around for a while. Eventually she pulled over into a gas station parking lot so we could talk some more, and I lost it. I cried my eyes out, probably not making any sense at all. She listened to me for a while, and when I was finished, there was silence. I asked, "What do you think I should do? Do you have any advice?" After a long pause, she said she wasn't sure. But she did have one piece of advice. I could tell she was nervous to share because it wasn't the advice I was wanting to hear, but she pressed on out of pure love for me. She told me something her mother had said to her throughout her whole life: simply say the name of Jesus. Renea explained that her mom did this all the time—when she knew what to do, but even more so when she didn't. She explained that there is power in the name of Jesus and that I didn't have to have the right words to pray or go through a checklist of things to make myself feel better. I just needed to draw near to Him and say His name.

Of course, she wasn't saying I *shouldn't* go to a doctor as well. She wasn't even saying I shouldn't be concerned or pray about it. She just wanted me to understand that there is power in Jesus's name, and when we don't know what else to do or say, His name is enough. I used her advice when getting an MRI for the headaches I had after my cancer treatments and it immediately calmed my nerves. Jesus was, and is, always with us. If this is the only thing you remember from this book, I believe reading it was still worth your time: when you don't know what to do—and even when you do—just say His name.

WE WILL OVERCOME

—JOSH AND ALY—

We have shared our story with others since Aly's initial cancer diagnosis on October 17, 2011. We've blogged, spoken in churches, been interviewed on the *Today Show*, on other television networks, in magazines and journals, and, of course, given America a front-row seat to our lives through *Rattled*. Through it all, people have asked us why we share so openly. There are many reasons why, but it all comes back to one *main* reason: we are overcomers. Revelation 12:11 says, "And they overcame him by the blood of the Lamb and by the word of their testimony" (NKJV). Those two separate, distinct parts—the blood of the Lamb and the word of their testimony—are so important, and we always want to be faithful to remember each one.

God has done so much in our life; He has poured out His love, grace, power, and healing more times than we can count. He was with us in the unfinished house when we first got the call that Aly had cancer. He was with us in Houston through all the treatments. He was with us throughout years of surgeries and reconstruction. He was with us through the trials and heartache of infertility. He was with us when Karen chose us to adopt Genevieve. He was with us when we got pregnant with Vera against all odds. He was with us when Karen's first instinct when she got pregnant again was to call us to adopt Lydia. He was with us as we celebrated five years cancer-free. God. Is. With. Us. Always and forever, He is with us. Our strength and our shield. Our Savior and Protector. Our Healer and Comforter. Our Lord and our God. He has given us everything, and we will shout the word of our testimony from the rooftops in honor and awe of what He has done.

So here's our challenge to you. Are you overcoming obstacles in your life? If you're not, why not? If you have accepted Jesus as the King of your life, you've got one part of the equation down. But don't skip the second part: your testimony. Share your story. Talk about what God has done, is doing, and will do in your life. It doesn't have to be a blog, a book, or a reality TV show, but do *something*. Share you story. Be open and vulnerable, even if it's just being honest with a group of friends about what's going on in your life. It's not enough to only *embrace* your story; you have to *share* it as well.

You've read our story.

We are Josh and Aly Taylor.

We are overcomers.

We are cancer survivors.

We are infertility conquerors.

We are blessed by adoption.

We are on a TV show.

We are cool with having our plans destroyed, because we know God's plans are better.

And we will never, never stop sharing what He has done.

Please determine to overcome and have your plans destroyed alongside us! We hope and pray you will invite Jesus into your life, genuinely ask Him to destroy your plans, and embrace the entirely *better* plans He has for you, even when you have no indication His plans are better. Trust us. Trust Him. They are. And once you discover that, share your incredible story about your plans being destroyed.

CHAPTER 15

LIFE-GIVING RESOURCES

—ALY—

During my cancer, infertility, adoption, and pregnancy journeys, there were many practical things that helped Josh and I get through each battle. I hope this section serves as a resource for you that you can turn to as you might fight a comparable battle to the ones we shared here, or you are wondering how to help someone who has fought a similar battle.

As you know well by now, I don't like the unknowns in life, and I so desired people to tell me what to do during my journey. Unfortunately, there weren't many "to dos," and that was an incredible lesson for me during my journey. Instead of the "to dos" I desperately desired, there was a lot of waiting and praying; however, there were things that helped me, and here is where I will share some of the most helpful and practical things Josh and I found during our journeys. I pray the things that helped me will help you too.

As we've walked this road, however, we've found that many people simply don't know what to do to support their friends and family members who have had their world rocked by a cancer diagnosis, a negative pregnancy test, failed fertility treatments, adoption struggles, and more. Every act of service was precious to us as we were fighting our battles, but honestly, not everything that came our way was helpful. We learned so much from our loved ones and we pray we can teach you a trick or two about how to care for those facing a devastating illness.

BE THE BODY OF CHRIST

Of all the wonderful gifts and acts of service our friends did for us during any of our battles, the thing that helped me the most were their prayers. If you tell someone you're going to pray for them, take it seriously. Go to battle for them. Fall on your knees before your heavenly Father for them. So often we tell people we'll pray for them and then either forget or just add their name to a one-time prayer list. Don't do that! Cancer patients are literally fighting for their lives; if you promise to pray for them, you're volunteering to serve the war effort!

For example, I often got texts in the middle of the night from people saying the Holy Spirit woke them up to pray for me. People like this— true prayer warriors—offered to pray for me, and then they'd come back to me later and tell me the *specific* things they prayed for. They proactively asked Josh and me what exactly they could pray for, what we were worried about, and what doctor appointments were coming up that week.

I remember going to bed so many nights nervous about whether I'd be able to sleep or not. I had so much on my mind, it was hard to truly relax and drift off to sleep. So Josh and I asked people to pray specifically for my sleep—and they did! Almost every night I'd get messages from prayer partners telling me they were praying for me to sleep soundly. One night a friend sent me this Scripture verse, which became dear to me throughout my battle: "When you lie down, you will not be afraid; when you lie down, your sleep will be sweet" (Proverbs 3:24). God is so good, and He answers His children's prayers!

Prayer Meetings

We told you earlier about the prayer-filled send-off party our friends and family gave us before we left for that first trip to Houston. I also had a different kind of prayer meeting around that same time. It was more like an intervention—they were intervening on my behalf to God for my healing. I was invited to my friends Margot and Ainsley's house. As I arrived, they immediately sat me on the couch and held my hands. I didn't know what was about to happen. They brought me a little white stapled book. I could tell it was a book full of scriptures. On the cover it had Matthew 18:19–20: "Again, truly I tell you that if two of you on earth agree about anything they ask for, it will be done for them by my Father in heaven. For where two or three gather in my name, there am I with them."

They sat with me for the next hour reading every scripture in the book, praying with me, and trusting with me that I was healed—that it had already been done. My job, then, was to walk out my journey in faith. This was the moment I truly started to understand what it meant to have people fighting your battles with and for you. These dear friends were not going to let me leave town without fully believing in my healing. They were willing to do whatever it took to give me hope and to fill me with faith in the Lord's healing power through Scripture. This is a picture of the body of Christ in action.

This same group of people always expected healing, and that positivity is desperately needed by people going through cancer. I remember how the people around me agonized and waited with me for news after every test, scan, and appointment. I needed people in those moments to fully expect me to be healed and remind me of Isaiah 53:5: "But He was wounded for our transgressions, He was bruised for our iniquities; the chastisement for our peace was upon Him, and by His stripes we are healed" (NKJV). It's hard to walk into a doctor's office and not know what news you're going to receive. It's a lot easier to face those conversations when the people around you feed your faith by saying things like, "Can't wait to hear the good results!" or "What an incredible testimony you will have!"

Mark 2 People

This same group of people prayed for us as we walked through our infertility and adoption journeys. As I stated earlier, we referred to these friends as our Mark 2 friends. We needed people to believe with us and have faith that what Jesus says in His Word will actually come to pass.

When I was going through infertility and did IVF (which you now know did not result in pregnancy), I sent out an email each day to my Mark 2 people, asking them to pray a specific prayer with us. I knew there was power in corporate prayer, and I needed faith-filled prayer like never before.

Here is an example of an email I sent out during my IVF. I called it my "Battle Plan."

Battle Plan Day 5
Friday, July 18, 2014
Stimulation Injections Start Today

My beginning injections have continued to go well. I have some bruising from the injections, but it really doesn't hurt much. It looks worse than it hurts. My two new stimulation drugs start today! So that will make 4 injections total a day. I am somewhat nervous about these . . . bigger needles, but these are the hard-core medications. And I am on the highest dosage possible on all medications. Apparently my ovaries will greatly increase in size, which could cause some pain and discomfort. But they are increased to make more eggs, so bring it on.

There are many steps to this process, but my doctor's main hope and concern is that we will have eggs to retrieve and then that they are of good quality. The blood test I had showed that was unlikely, but we are believing differently. So lots of eggs and good quality eggs are *huge* for me and us making a baby!

Prayer points:

- These new medications help me produce more eggs than the doctors expect.
- The eggs produced will be of perfect quality and they will be able to retrieve plenty of them.
- That we put our faith in God, not totally in these medications. He alone is the author of life.
- That God will increase our faith and for fear to leave. We want excitement and expectation to take over.
- That we don't have any trouble in administering injections.
- That I will have no adverse side effects to this medication. That my ovaries will not have any adverse long-term harmful effects.
- That Josh and I will be given wisdom as this process begins. We need clear guidance on how to proceed with this process.
- That God will provide for us financially as we begin this expensive process.

Scripture to Personally Confess:

"Children are a gift from the LORD;
    they are a reward from him.
Children born to [Aly and Josh]
    are like arrows in a warrior's hands.
How joyful [are Aly and Josh] whose quiver is full of them!
    [They] will not be put to shame when [they confront their] accusers at the city gates."
—Psalm 127:3–5 (NLT)

Confession to Pray:

> "Father, no plague, no evil shall come near Josh and Aly's dwelling. Aly is healed by the stripes of Jesus. Sickness of any kind is taken out of her midst. You said ask anything of You in Jesus's name and it would be done; and that if two of us on earth agree on anything it would be done. So we pray and agree with You and Your word, Father, that Aly and Josh will conceive and bring forth a healthy, precious baby to Your glory and honor."

You may wonder, *Wow, that is amazing! But, Aly, you didn't get pregnant with IVF. Your so-called "battle plan" did not work.* Yes, what we were praying and believing for didn't happen like we thought it would. But, man, did our faith grow like never before. And, as you know now, God did give us what we believed for in His perfect timing, not ours. As we prayed the same prayers and walked through each day together, God moved. And once we learned I wasn't pregnant, we trusted in His will and His timing.

Faith builds faith, and having others help build my faith with their own gave me new strength, kept my hope alive, and transformed my attitude. With friends like that, I couldn't help but believe I was healed. If you know others are walking through cancer or another terrible illness, I strongly encourage you to speak life to them. Be the hope and encouragement they need. Help keep their faith alive by pouring your faith into them!

LEND YOUR EXPERTISE
AND OFFER SPECIFIC HELP

—JOSH—

When Aly was diagnosed, I quickly realized how much I hadn't done to help other people going through that kind of nightmare. Sure, I was only twenty-seven at the time, but there's still so much I could have done to be a blessing to the hurting people in my community. Going forward, Aly and I made a commitment to serve others however we could, whether it's in big or small ways. Fortunately, the people in our life stepped up and modeled what that kind of loving care and service can look like.

One of the biggest blessings we received came soon after Aly's initial diagnosis. We mentioned earlier in the book that we were in the process of building a house at the time, and we were doing a lot of the work ourselves to save money. Obviously, once we learned Aly had cancer, everything stopped on the house. I couldn't imagine wasting an ounce of energy or effort on the house when my wife needed all I had to offer. She was my priority; the house could wait.

A couple of weeks after we got the news about Aly's cancer, our friend, Jonathan, approached me and asked if he could help finish the house for us. That would have been a great offer from anyone, but this guy happens to be one of the best contractors in town. He wasn't just offering to swing a hammer for us; he was offering his full expertise as a contractor to finish our home. I can't tell you what this meant to me. My friend, seeing this very specific need—and knowing he was specifically equipped to meet it—stepped in. As a result, we ended up with a much nicer house than we would have had if I had done all the work myself. With my friend's help (along with the help of our neighbors and church family) our house was ready just after Christmas that year!

—ALY—

Another thing that helped us tremendously was getting help on *specific* things. I learned through my cancer journey that it's hard for me to accept help from people. People always said, "Let me know if I can do anything," or "What can I do to help?" Almost every time early on, I'd reply, "Oh, we're good, but thanks!" Or I'd tell them I'd let them know if I thought of something—but then never did. What a waste! I had a whole community of people around me who wanted to help; all I had to do was give them some direction on *how* to help—but I didn't do it.

However—and this is key—I realized I was a lot more comfortable accepting people's help when they offered something specific. If someone said, "What do you need?" I couldn't tell them. It felt too much like an imposition. But if they said, "Give me your grocery list; I'm going to the store for you," I didn't hesitate to let them help. Other times someone might say, "I'm bringing you guys dinner tonight. What do you want?" There's so much freedom in that kind of offer, because you aren't putting the burden of the request on the sick person. Instead, you're taking the initiative to identify a specific need and proactively telling them you're going to meet it.

I'd also encourage you to marry this specific need-meeting with what I call the *front porch concept*. When I was going through chemo and radiation and recovering from surgery, I didn't want to see anyone. I felt terrible and usually didn't feel like painting a smile on my face for someone. That's when I realized how much I appreciated the people who just dropped off stuff at my front door. A friend would get a few things at the store for me, put them on my porch, and leave without ringing the bell. I can't tell you how loved I felt when I got a text that said something like, "Hey, Aly! I just dropped off a bag of groceries for you. They're on your porch right now. Love you!" It seems so simple, but it's an amazing expression of love not only to take care of someone's needs but to also be so thoughtful.

Don't just ask people what you can do for them; *find out* what you can do for them. Identify the specific things they need help with and try to make a huge impact in one particular area. That's the kind of help that really makes a life-changing difference to someone in need.

GIVE MONEY AND RESOURCES

—JOSH—

We've told you how our friends and community came around us to help meet our specific needs, but I want to be super clear on this: there is no possible way we would have survived financially if it were not for the generosity of others during our fight with cancer, infertility, and adoption. We would have had to move in with our parents just to try to stay afloat. Before Aly's cancer diagnosis, I had recently left my coaching job, and it was now clear to me why God put that surprising call on my heart: He freed up more of my time to spend with Aly during those years of treatment and surgery. That meant, though, that we had lost a big part of our income.

On top of that, I took off a ton of time from my other job at the school to be with Aly as much as possible for all her appointments and recovery. Thankfully, insurance covered most of Aly's medical bills, but there was still a surprising amount of out-of-pocket expenses for different tests and medicines during cancer and infertility. And then there was all the travel. We were on the road all the time driving to and from Houston and then back and forth to Jackson, Mississippi during Aly's fertility treatments. I've already said that I have some anxiety around finances, so believe me when I say my "provider" nerve was twitching quite often.

I can't count how many times, though, that money would appear out of nowhere. One time, for example, Aly had to have a breast cancer genetic test that cost $2,500, and we were devastated to learn our insurance wouldn't cover it. The next day we received a check in the mail for that exact amount from a friend. He didn't know anything about the genetic test; he was just being generous and faithful to God's call to give. We know it was really God who put those checks in our mailbox right when we needed them, but He did that through generous people. We even had an incredibly dear and generous friend give us money each week for five years. Five years! We felt so undeserving and asked her to stop. She was adamant that God had put this on her heart and would keep on giving until He moved her heart towards another need. We could never thank all of them enough for supporting us financially during the darkest days of our life.

—ALY—

People blew us away with their generosity. People helped us in many ways, financially and otherwise. Someone once paid for our rental cars while traveling, another friend gave us a gas card to use for traveling to and from Houston for each treatment, my mom let us use her car to drive to Houston and offered to be with me 24-7 if need be, my mother-in-law made and delivered to me a fresh smoothie or juice every morning, people went out of their way to make cancer-fighting foods for me, and people sent us grocery gift cards. Some friends even personally flew us to one of my treatments in a private plane!

Amazing things happen when people open their hearts and wallets *and* try to find the specific things you really need. There were many times that our friends noticed a need that we hadn't even considered yet. What a blessing to have a need met before it ever became an issue for us. The outpouring of love and support we received over those years has encouraged us to dig deep into how we can really serve someone who needs help. We don't settle for, "I'll let you know if I think of anything." Instead, we get involved and try to find a specific thing to do for someone or buy for them.

BE A GATEKEEPER

—JOSH—

When Aly was going through her treatments and word spread that she had cancer, we found that people started crawling out of the woodwork to tell us their cancer stories. Some of them were good, encouraging accounts of how God healed them or their loved ones. Others, though, were crazy nightmare stories about the absolute worst things you can imagine. So many people came up to us and told us their cancer horror stories that I quickly nominated myself to be Aly's gatekeeper. Remember, we didn't even want the doctors sharing unnecessary statistics with us, and we had sworn off reading scary stories on the internet; we certainly didn't want to hear a hopeless stranger speculate on the worst things that might happen.

I got pretty good at sniffing out the people who wanted to tell Aly about their aunt who passed away from breast cancer or a cousin who had a bad surgery experience. When we were going through fertility treatments, many times people would come up to Aly to share about a miscarriage or stillbirth. Then, it seemed to be even worse when we made the decision to adopt. I could point people out who were determined to tell me the struggles they were having with children they adopted and the "issues" we might face. I by no means am saying that their concerns were not valid or pure, but there were times where hearing that discouraging information just wasn't helpful. Whenever I saw them coming, I jumped in and derailed the conversation or flat-out blocked them from getting to my wife. Sometimes that meant they had to tell *me* the story. As much as I didn't want to hear about their negative experiences, I *definitely* didn't want Aly to have to listen to them. So if you're close to someone facing cancer, infertility, adoption, or a miracle pregnancy that could lend its way to fear, volunteer to be that person's gatekeeper. If you're the patient's spouse, good news: it's *already* your job!

And now a word for the rest of you: Please think before you speak. I don't want to be harsh, but it's never appropriate to tell a cancer patient the dark details of your long lost loved one who died from cancer. It rarely helps to tell someone who is fighting infertility about recurrent miscarriages. It never helps to tell someone considering adoption of all the horror stories. I know it hurts and you might feel a special connection to someone who's fighting the same battle you've been through, but many times, your story will do them more harm than good. Now, there is a time and place to share stories in order to help us process and move forward emotionally, but these stories are best for a group or therapy environment. When someone is fighting for her life or trying to create a life, she needs to hear positive, affirming, life-giving stories. She doesn't need you speaking death or negativity into her life.

And if I may be so bold, she also doesn't need you questioning her medical decisions. This one surprised and hurt Aly and me. We carefully considered and thoroughly prayed over her cancer treatment and fertility options. It was often agonizing trying to figure out which doctor's opinion to go with and which option would work best. Then, when we made those hard decisions, we were shocked to have people question everything we were doing or try to change our minds. We chose early on to listen to only positive voices and to cut out those who spoke death or second-guessed all our treatment plans.

If you truly want to be a source of hope for someone going through cancer, infertility, or adoption, take a good look at what you're saying and why you're saying it. Oftentimes it's better just to keep quiet. And simply offering to pray together may be the biggest blessing you can give over sharing a story or an opinion.

BECOMING A HEALTHY FOODIE

—ALY—

When I was initially diagnosed with cancer, I became strangely preoccupied with food. Okay, the truth is *obsessed* is probably a more accurate description—but not in the way you might think. I was scared to eat anything. I knew I had cancer growing in my body, and I didn't know what might make the cancer better or worse. As a result, I didn't eat much of anything for a while. I started reading and researching everything I could find on diet and cancer-fighting foods. There was so much I *couldn't* do in the healing process, so I was determined to control as much of it as I could. So I studied. And studied. And studied and studied and studied. I felt like I couldn't eat *anything* until I had it all figured out.

One night Josh and I were in his old bedroom at his parents' house when his mom knocked on the door. Through tears, she told me she wanted to help me with my diet. She said she'd start researching and helping me with anything related to food. I hugged and thanked her, and she left the room. As soon as the door closed, I buried my face in a pillow and burst into tears. That was the first time I really understood how much of a monster I'd turned the food issue into. But now I had a partner, someone who had seen this specific need and volunteered to help with it. I can't tell you what a relief it was to get help with this.

Changing my diet was a huge shift from what I ate pre-cancer. It was not as though all I ate was junk food; however, living in the South, we value good southern cooking, and I love all the good foods—pasta, pizza, Mexican, ice cream, sweets . . . all the healthy foods, of course. Before cancer, I always associated being "healthy" with my weight. Any time I would attempt to eat healthy it was always a motivation to lose weight. It was never really about filling my body with foods that would make me strong. So this undertaking of changing my diet was literally a 180 degree turnaround!

I do believe that God gave us so many natural things to keep us healthy and strong. I know He desires for me to be healthy—He designed my body as His temple, and I am committed to taking care of it. 1 Corinthians 6:19–20 tells us, "Do you not know that your bodies are temples of the Holy Spirit, who is in you, whom you have received from God? You are not your own; you were bought at a price. Therefore honor God with your bodies." This mind-set for my body has been one of the biggest lifestyle changes for me. One that has affected my husband and a lifestyle that I hope and pray to raise our children up in. I desire for them to live long, healthy lives as well!

What I am sharing with you is not an "anti-cancer" diet or even foods that can cure cancer, but simply diet choices that I've made to help me get and stay as healthy as possible. I have dreams one day of writing a cookbook!

Basic Restrictions

- Little to no bread. If I ever eat bread, I will do whole wheat or whole wheat tortillas.
- Little to no sugar. I try to stay away from sugar totally, outside of fruits and other foods with naturally occurring sugar.
- No cream or dairy products. I do eat eggs and drink unsweetened vanilla almond milk.
- No red meat, except for venison (deer meat), as it is very lean. As deer meat may not be for everyone, turkey is another great alternative to beef.
- I try to stay away from all processed food. If I do eat something processed, I try to eat organically.

Foods That Fill

- Oatmeal
- Organic cereals with little sugar
- Eggs, fish, chicken, or venison
- Veggies and fruits
- Brown rice
- Unsweetened vanilla almond milk
- Fresh juices
- Nuts (mainly almonds and walnuts)
- Sweet potatoes
- Raisins
- Lots of salad greens
- Avocado
- Black beans
- KIND bars or Lärabars
- Almond butter
- Unsweetened coconut milk
- Olive oil
- Honey and stevia for sweeteners

I've read blogs that say that eating healthy is just as costly as eating unhealthy, and I just haven't found that to be the case. It is so much more expensive, at least for us. Our grocery bill has nearly tripled each month since my diet changes. It is just one of the many sacrifices we make, and I have to see it as an investment. Being as frugal as we are, it is painful at times to see that money going to food and a gym membership! But I have to remind myself that it is an investment in my family's health and, ultimately, our lives.

BEWARE OF (SOME) BOOKS

Books are often the go-to gift when you don't know what to give someone who's just received bad news or is heading into a scary time of life. But be super careful here. I'll be the first to admit that I love research. It's hard to complete a PhD without fostering a healthy love of books!

As you know from reading the introduction to this book, one of our motivations for writing this book was the lack of hopeful books written by young girls like me with my type of breast cancer. For the most part, I received some incredible, inspirational books on healing. But then, there were a few books given to me that were amazing stories about a life well lived during cancer, but sadly that person fighting ended up passing away. It wasn't what I needed to read when I was praying, trusting, and believing I would live.

Instead, I chose to surround myself with books on healing. I wanted to read stories of real people with grim diagnoses who were alive today. It's surprising how few of those books are out there. That's honestly a big reason Josh and I decided to write *this* book. We want to show people that miracles happen, that healing is real, and that there are plenty of cancer survivors in the world. I'm honored to lend my voice to that incredible group of heroes, and I wish more survivors would raise their hands, tell their stories, and (even better) write more books.

The same caution applies when buying a book about infertility. Instead of all the statistics, find stories of those who overcame odds and became pregnant. Be careful when buying adoption books too. Instead of buying books on struggles that parents and children can sometimes go through when they experience adoption, buy the books that show the beauty of adoption and the incredible parallel it is for how God has adopted us. He literally sees us and Jesus the same. We are both His children—how incredible is that?

Chances are, people don't need you to add more ideas to their research pile. Instead, choose life-giving, hopeful stories about people who survived. You could also give them a book on healing, a Bible, or a devotional. The word *cancer, infertility,* or *adoption* doesn't even have to be on the cover!

RECOMMENDED BOOKS, BLOGS, SOCIAL MEDIA, AND WEBSITES

Books and blogs near and dear to my heart during our battles include:

- *Healed of Cancer* by Dodie Osteen
- *Hannah's Hope* by Jennifer Saake
- Unceasinglove.com
- Faithfuladoptionconsultants.com
- Christianadoptionconsultants.com

BE THERE CONSISTENTLY

—JOSH—

Perhaps the most important piece of advice I can give you as you seek to serve and love your hurting friends is to be there *consistently*. Every gift is meaningful, and we will always be grateful for every gift, card, prayer, and act of service anyone sent our way. There are a handful of people who walked with us each day and became a constant, steady source of encouragement and support for us.

The most astounding thing anyone did for us throughout Aly's whole cancer journey was the simplest thing in the world: someone sent Aly cards. That doesn't seem like a huge deal, but a lovely woman named Jody mailed Aly a card *every day for an entire year*. Can you imagine what it was like for my wife to walk to the mailbox each day to find a card from Jody? It wasn't much; she simply wrote a scripture on the card and told Aly that she prayed that scripture over her that day. That's the kind of thing most people would do once or twice, but this wonderful woman of God did it *every day*. What an encouragement! What an incredible act of love to show that kind of ongoing commitment and partnership.

The really cool thing about this is that Jody wasn't one of our close friends. When she started sending cards, I'd say Jody was an acquaintance at best. She's been part of our community for a few years, but we never dreamed God would work through her to make such a profound impact on Aly's life during her recovery. Today, all these years later, we have every scripture this lady sent us framed and hanging on the wall of our home as a reminder to care for others and that God's Word never fails.

If you really want to make a difference in someone's toughest times, be there consistently. Stand in the trenches with that person every day. Even if it's just a daily prayer, a text, a phone call, a Facebook post, or whatever else you choose, find some way to make an ongoing impact on a struggling person's life. Make sure that person knows you're not just going to be there *once*, but *always*.

BE THERE IN THE AFTERMATH

—ALY—

This chapter has covered many specific ways the people around us loved and served us during our fight with cancer, infertility, and adoption, but I think the most important and most helpful thing to us was that people *kept* giving and doing this for us after the so-called "battle" was won. I was so naïve before I went through cancer. I thought that once people became cancer-free, their lives were great and they no longer needed all the support they'd received during their sickest days. Wow, was I wrong. I needed more support *after* cancer than I did *during*! And this was true with infertility and adoption too.

I'm not so naïve about this stuff anymore. Now I know the aftermath of cancer, infertility, and adoption is real, and I maintain my support of others long after their chemo and radiation are done. I maintain support for those who are still trying to grow their families. I maintain support for those who have walked the miraculous road of adoption. It's hard to understand, but there is a certain burden to being cancer-free, and we often needed others to help us carry that load. As the Bible says, we should "carry each other's burdens, and in this way [we] will fulfill the law of Christ" (Galatians 6:2). So my final encouragement to you my friends, as a "burden bearer," is to stick with people long after the treatments and surgeries are done. Help them readjust to their new lives as cancer survivors. Be there to celebrate their two-year, five-year, sixty-year cancer-free milestones. Stick with the person who continues to cry after each negative pregnancy test. Stick with the person who still mourns a miscarriage or stillbirth. Stick with the person who goes through the adoption process and needs love, prayers, and support. All of my difficult life experiences have shown me in vivid color who my true friends and family members are, and our relationships—and my life—will always be richer for it.

ACKNOWLEDGEMENTS

There are so many people who contributed to the writing of this book. We realize that telling what all the amazing people in our lives mean to us and what they have done for us would be an entire other book in itself. We are continually blown away by God's goodness to us, and one of the main ways we see His goodness is through people who have been placed in our lives for such a time as this. They are His hands and feet on earth glorifying His kingdom.

We want to thank our parents (Cyd, Joey, Renea, and Terry) most of all, as they have held our hands and hearts through our cancer, infertility, adoption, and pregnancy journeys. If not for their prayers, support, and sacrifices, I guarantee you this book would not have been a reality. To our parents: We could never say thank you enough for all you do for us daily. We love you. And we are so thankful to have parents who we love and like. We are so blessed to do life with you.

A tremendous thank you to our precious family and friends who have walked through our trials right alongside of us. Jessica, Jeremy J., Lee, Rachel, Ainsley, Margot, Kelly, Kase, Katie, Kyle, Ashley, Richard R., Jr., Angie, Jonathan, Tara, Tammy, Mel, Marty, Lance, Jenny, Jason H., Alicia, Erin, Case, Jeff, Brenda, Ron S., Ryan, Kimmie, Lindsay, Jeremy S., Lindsey, Andrea, Jason I., Matt, Kristen, Kitty, Casey, Ann S., James, Larry, Julie C., Bebee, Ann G., Doug, Jake, Sherry, Cathy, Rhonda, Hank, Darren, Candace, Brandon B., Julie B., Tara, Drew, Ron H., Amy, Lauren, Jana F., Chris, Georgiana, Brandon T., Sonja, John, Megan, Jayson, Christi,

Michael, Beck, Jodi, Richard R. Sr., Sherie, Arvil, Cheryl, Michelle, Eddie, Jana C., Brooke, Micah, Alison, Randy, Julie V., Andy, Vasoula, Beth, Patti, Lonnie, Roseann, and Clint: You held our arms up when we had no strength. We love you with all our hearts.

A special thanks goes to the publishing team at Worthy, who have been amazing to work with. Thank you Leeanna, Allen, and Julie for helping us structure this book to be what we envisioned it to be. Thank you for putting our tangled thoughts into beautiful words that conveyed our hearts perfectly. And to our "unofficial" editor: Mom, thank you for all your hard work and for reading every draft, even when I couldn't begin to read your hand writing.

Another special thank you goes to TLC and Magilla productions for believing in our story and recognizing that it was one the world needed to hear and see. Thank you for showing us as we are, warts and all. Thank you for giving us the freedom to share our faith and capturing some of the most incredible moments of our lives.

To John and Chrys Howard: Thank you for believing in us. Thank you for your prayers, words of wisdom, and help in making this book a reality. We are forever indebted for your time, love, and advice to us. We love you.

To all of the hotel lobbies this book was written in, thank you. A bonus piece of advice: if you are ever needing a quiet space to write, think, or just be, go to your local hotel lobby. You won't run into anyone you know, and you have all the amenities. Best. Idea. Ever.

It goes without saying, but our adoration and thankfulness to God has never been greater. Jesus: Thank You for allowing this book to happen. Thank You for turning our mourning into dancing, and giving us this platform to share Your glory more and more with the world. This book is called *Aly's Fight*, but as You know, the fight was all Yours. And it's been won. We are living in victory, Jesus. Glory and honor to You, forever and ever.

ABOUT THE AUTHORS

ALY TAYLOR is a grateful wife of one amazing man and a mom of three toddlers. She can be found most days still in her robe and slippers by lunch time. Aly is a full-time homemaker and it is the greatest joy in her life to be able to stay home with her children.

During naptime, Aly is an adjunct professor for Liberty University, adoption consultant and homestudy provider, speaker, and family therapist. Aly received her PhD during her breast cancer battle, and loves that she can help others from the comfort of her own home.

Aly enjoys writing, reading, doing anything adventurous or outside, snow skiing, exercising, laughing uncontrollably with her husband and friends, taking naps (though rare and far between), traveling, and having dance parties with her little family. Aly finds joy in each day and realizes what a gift it is to wake up and be able to breathe. She always says that "a bad day is still a good day." Through her cancer journey, she learned that any day alive is a good day, and she strives to live by that each day.

JOSH TAYLOR is a man who is still in awe that he gets to spend time with his four miracle girls every day. Waking up with Aly and going to get their three little girls out of their beds each morning is the joy of his life. Josh is a serial entrepreneur who loves real estate and tackling new ideas and projects; however, he strives to not be known by what he does, but who he is.

Josh works as a contractor for his business, J. TaylorMade Construction. For him, building homes, renovating, and watching something transform is an incredibly rewarding thing to be a part of. Josh also does real estate, including buying, selling, and renting properties.

He also loves speaking with Aly all over the country, and continues to mentor men—his greatest passion outside of his family.

Josh enjoys spending time outdoors, bow hunting, fishing, snow skiing, and laughing with Aly and friends. He thrives off of friendships that aren't the typical "man" friendships, but the ones that are raw and real. After a long day of managing projects, his favorite part of the day is coming home to his little girls running to see him and embracing Aly.

JOSH AND ALY have been married for almost 13 years and live in West Monroe, Louisiana raising their three girls, Genevieve, Vera, and Lydia. They live in a neighborhood with some of their best friends and parents right down the road. They firmly believe in the phrase, "it takes a village!" They have a 12-year-old chocolate lab, their first baby, Bella. They travel the country sharing their story of healing, hope, and miracles. They strive to live each day abundantly and center their marriage and home around the life-changing power of Jesus Christ.

You can find us sharing stories of great people or companies helping those facing numerous types of battles, inspirational content, as well as stories of our lives daily.

- Alysfight.com
- Instagram: @alysfight
- Facebook: facebook.com/alysfight
- Twitter: @alyptaylor and @JoshTaylorLa

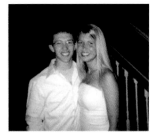

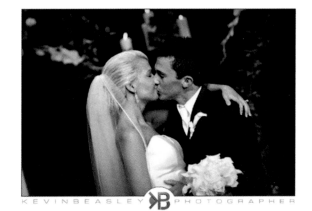

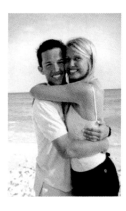

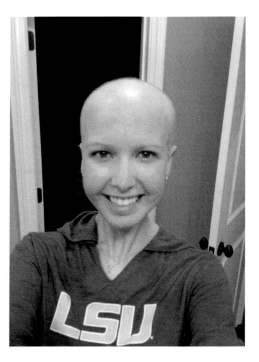

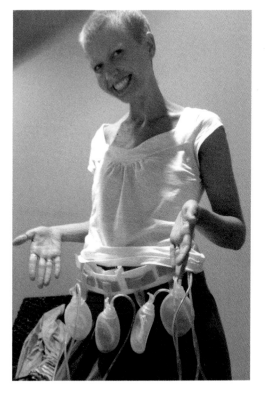

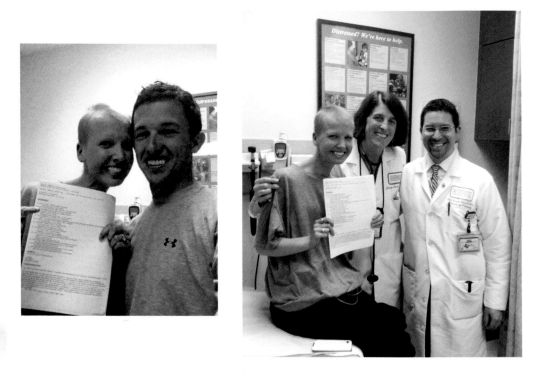

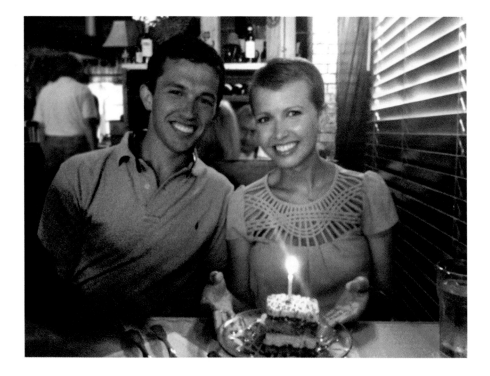

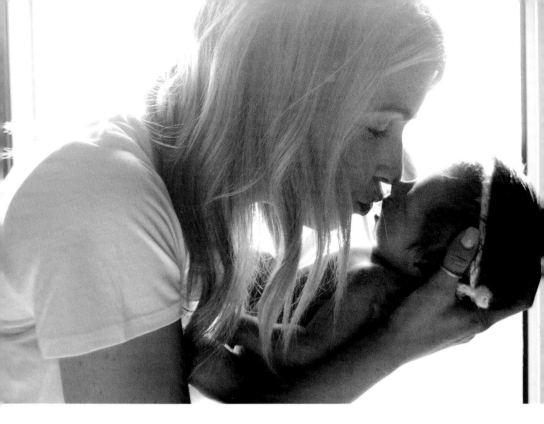

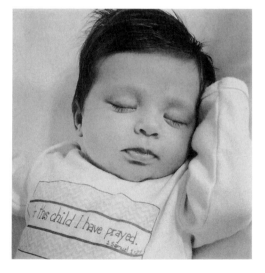

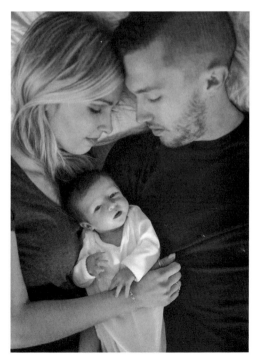

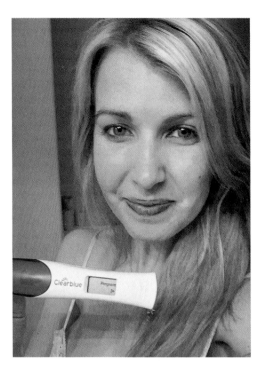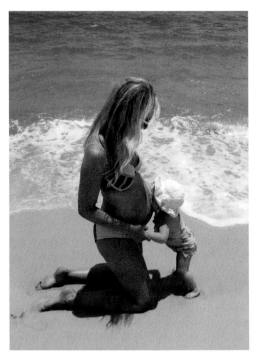

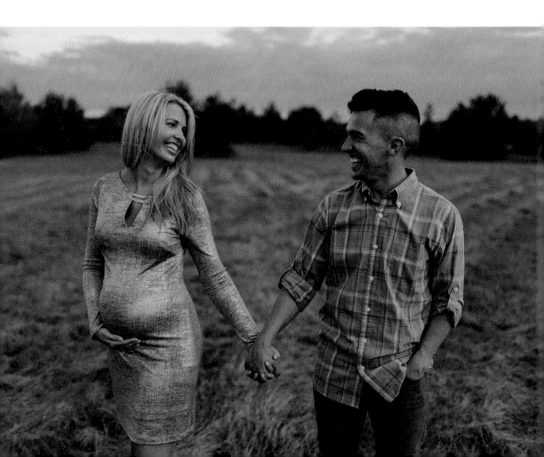

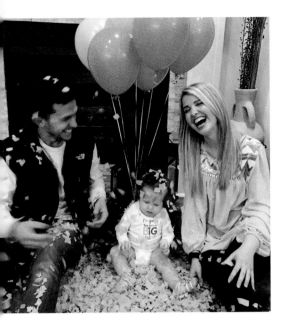
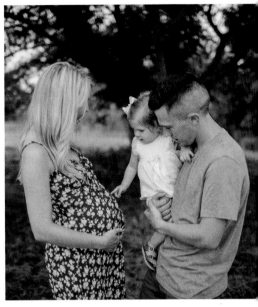
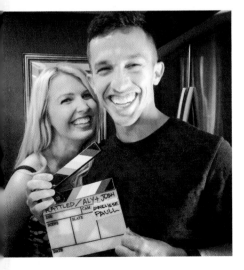
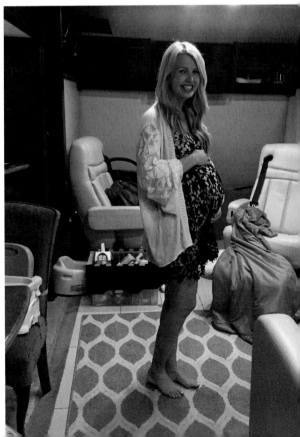

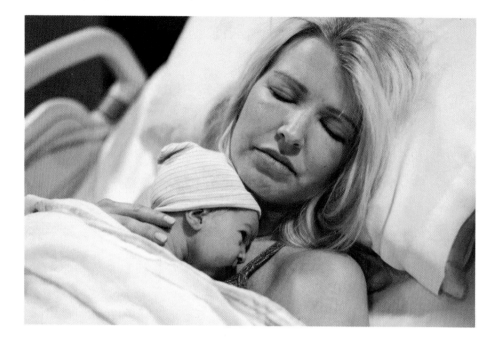

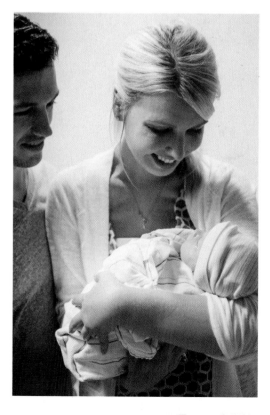

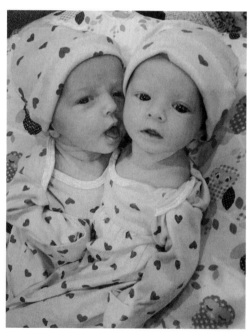

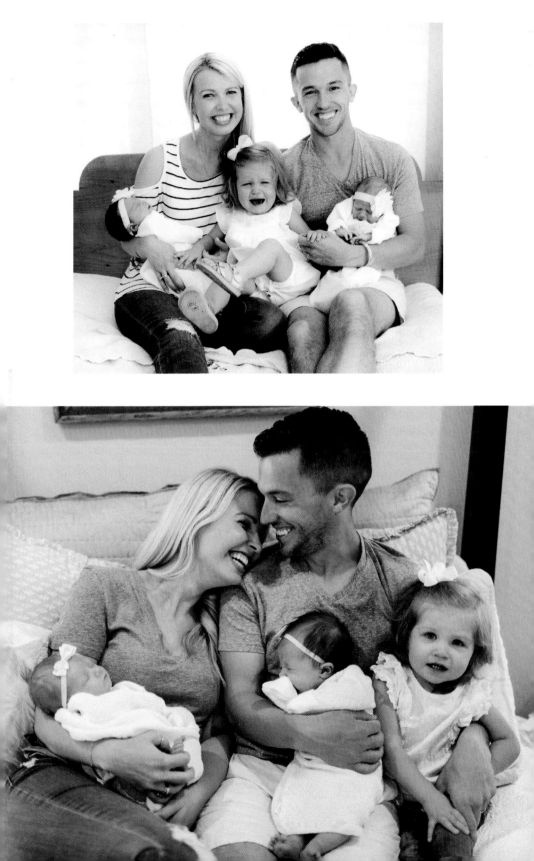

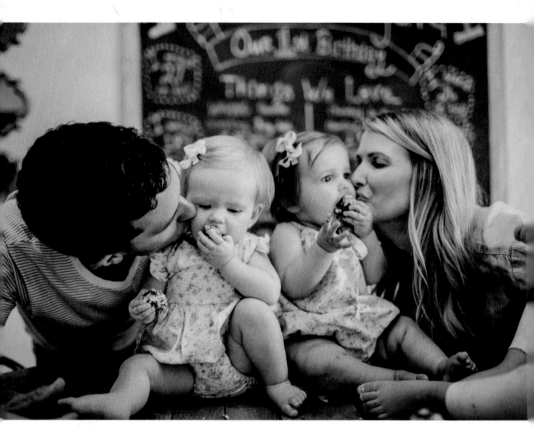

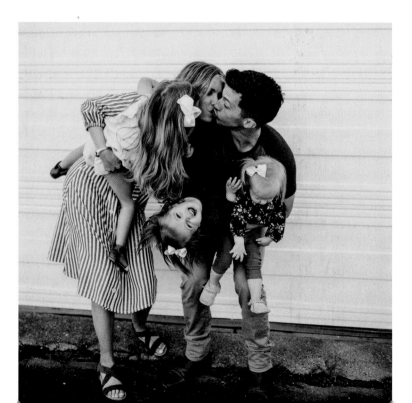